Strength and Conditioning Coaching
Winning Methods, Programs, and Facilities

Strength and Conditioning Coaching
Winning Methods, Programs, and Facilities

Michael Boyle

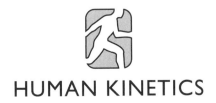

HUMAN KINETICS

Library of Congress Cataloging-in-Publication Data

Library of Congress Cataloging-in-Publication information is available. LCCN 2025007618 (print).

ISBN: 978-1-7182-4584-6 (print)

Copyright © 2026, 2023 by Michael John Boyle

Human Kinetics supports copyright. Copyright fuels scientific and artistic endeavor, encourages authors to create new works, and promotes free speech. Thank you for buying an authorized edition of this work and for complying with copyright laws by not reproducing, scanning, or distributing any part of it in any form without written permission from the publisher. You are supporting authors and allowing Human Kinetics to continue to publish works that increase the knowledge, enhance the performance, and improve the lives of people all over the world.

To report suspected copyright infringement of content published by Human Kinetics, contact us at **permissions@hkusa. com**. To request permission to legally reuse content published by Human Kinetics, please refer to the information at **https:// US.HumanKinetics.com/pages/permissions-translations-faqs**.

This publication is written and published to provide accurate and authoritative information relevant to the subject matter presented. It is published and sold with the understanding that the author and publisher are not engaged in rendering legal, medical, or other professional services by reason of their authorship or publication of this work. If medical or other expert assistance is required, the services of a competent professional person should be sought.

This book is a revised edition of *Designing Strength Training Programs and Facilities, Second Edition*, published in 2023 by On Target Publications.

Human Kinetics books are available at special discounts for bulk purchase. Special editions or book excerpts can also be created to specification. For details, contact the Special Sales Manager at Human Kinetics.

Printed in the United States of America   10 9 8 7 6 5 4 3 2 1

Human Kinetics
1607 N. Market Street
Champaign, IL 61820
USA

United States and International
Website: US.HumanKinetics.com
Email: info@hkusa.com
Phone: 1-800-747-4457

Canada
Website: Canada.HumanKinetics.com
Email: info@hkcanada.com

Human Kinetics' authorized representative for product safety in the EU is Mare Nostrum Group B.V., Mauritskade 21D, 1091 GC Amsterdam, The Netherlands.
Email: gpsr@mare-nostrum.co.uk

L1352

IN APPRECIATION

Thanks to the following people for the great photos in this book.

Photos by Ben Connolly

Athlete Models

Bre Gustin

Courtney Moulton

Cam McGhee

Lauren Martuscello

Steve Bigelow

CONTENTS

Acknowledgments	9
Foreword by Dan John	11
Preface	13
Introduction	15
Chapter 1—Designing and Equipping Your Facility	21
Chapter 2—Building a Strong Program Foundation	29
Chapter 3—Designing the Perfect Program	33
Chapter 4—Core Training, Mobility, Activation and Warm-Ups	43
Chapter 5—Explosive Training	59
Chapter 6—Strength Training	69
Chapter 7—Lower-Body Training	73
Chapter 8—Upper-Body Pulling and Pressing	105
Chapter 9—Choosing a System of Training	113
Chapter 10—Creating Efficient and Effective Workouts	123
Chapter 11—Speed Development	133
Chapter 12—Conditioning	149
Chapter 13—Computerizing Your Program	161
Chapter 14—Designing Programs for Teams or Groups	165
Chapter 15—Parting Words: The Mirror and the Window	173
Recommended Reading	175
References	177
Index	179
About the Author	187
Earn Continuing Education Credits/Units	189

ACKNOWLEDGMENTS

In the acknowledgments of *Functional Training for Sports,* I thanked many people who were influential in my development as a coach. As I rewrite this, my second book, I realize some people are responsible for my development as both a coach and as a person. I want to thank those who made it possible for me to think, write and speak. There are far too many to list, so I won't try.

However, I'd be remiss if I didn't mention Chris Poirier. He's long been a friend, an advisor and a huge Mike Boyle/Mike Boyle Strength and Conditioning supporter.

It's still a joy to do something I love every day, and for this I'm truly grateful.

Cindy, Michaela and Mark help me realize it's not about money or fame, but about being with people I love.

FOREWORD

DAN JOHN

"At the time, I thought I was clever, but I now realize I was very dumb."

Mike Boyle remains one of the best and sanest voices in the fitness field. In a field filled with bunk science, junk information and charlatans, Mike's sound and grounded insights and observations keep us on the right path. This little line, "At the time, I thought I was clever, but I now realize I was very dumb," summarizes the genius we find when we interact with Mike. He uses his experience to inform his logic and his logic to inform his experience.

Whenever I read his work or listen to him on podcasts or from the stage at Perform Better, I'm dropped into the deep end of ongoing practice and reasoning. Unlike the vacuous minions of social media experts who prod and push us to the sexy new ideas and exotic elixirs, Mike trains actual athletes and actual human beings and makes them ready for elite sport and life achievement.

He does something few do: He changes his mind. He listens and learns. He adapts. He has the odd capacity to admit mistakes…a skill many of us should learn. It's rare. It's rare in our times that an expert—and Mike is clearly an expert—will have the brutal honesty to say both "I was right" and "I was wrong." Both statements, by the way, are difficult to admit when one reviews a multi-decade career at the top of a field.

Mike's new book, *Strength and Conditioning Coaching*, sits us down in the first row of the classroom. Sit up straight and keep your pen ready. Every page finds a new insight, a new answer. Mike questions just about everything we do in the world of strength and conditioning and logically leads us to a conclusion. Disagree as you wish, but be sure you understand the discussion before you wade in to the deep waters here.

In the middle of the book, Mike presents a detailed discussion about popular training programs that dominated the early years of the Wild, Wild West, also known as the "internet." Certainly, history has taught us that religious wars can be the worst—the internet wars over one set to failure versus Olympic lifts to failure have cost many friendships and produced many injuries. Mike offers us a better way:

"Having knowledge is one thing. Being able to take that knowledge and use it to design a program is another thing entirely. The key to being able to design great training programs is the ability to filter information. You can't make big program changes every time a new idea comes across your desk. You need to look at the new information and then filter out the hype."

"Filter information."

If you need a two-word summary for this book for your review, there you go. This is Mike's great strength (Ha! He's a strength coach): He has that ability to receive information, study a trend and squeeze out the material that's reasonable, appropriate and doable for his clients and athletes and to pass along to coaches.

There are dozens of points in this book where I think, "Hey, I do that!" Hopefully, most of the time, it's a positive thing, but like most of us, Gentle Reader, I tend to be on the idiot side of Mike's point. Like many hard-driving coaches, I pushed exhausted athletes to more exhaustion. Ideally, I've learned from those mistakes.

Mike comforts us as he lets us know that "doing something" gives our athletes and our programs a "slight edge."

Success in sports, and also in life, is often simply doing the little things right when the coach or Mom isn't watching.

And if you need proof of Mike's insights on taking athletes to the next level with that "slight edge," simply read the section on sprinting in the weightroom. I remain stunned at how Mike has knitted the best and brightest of track and field into success with sprints surrounded by platforms, racks and plates.

This book is a master course in looking at the little things. If you're stacking the walls with a bunch of squat racks, a few minutes of math will save you hours of issues later...including moving literally tons of equipment back and forth across the room.

And if you find a new exercise—and good for you—spend a few minutes of thinking about which "old" exercises to drop, adapt or discard.

Mike Boyle is the coach coaches need. This book is the sum of decades of his experience and insight.

Read this book. Devour this book.

And become a better coach, athlete and trainer from your time reading Mike Boyle.

Dan John

PREFACE

This is the book I always wanted to write. It's a serious strength training manual for coaches who want to get the most out of their athletes. My first book, *Functional Training for Sports,* was a more mainstream piece intended for athletes, coaches and trainers. While *Functional Training for Sports* was a success, I also wanted to write a book for serious strength and conditioning professionals I consider to be my peers.

In this version of the book, I'll intentionally not go into great detail about areas I covered in *Functional Training for Sports* or in the second edition, *New Functional Training for Sports.* I'm updating this text to represent my current views.

There's a great deal of new and updated material here, yet at times parts from the original book are repeated so the text flows well. You may have read some of this before, but I made every effort to update all sections.

The focus of this book is on how to put together a program. My goal is for this to be the type of book I coveted in my early years of coaching, much like *The Charlie Francis Training System* (now called *Training for Speed*) and Bill Starr's *The Strong Shall Survive* hold those places of importance in my mind. Those works formed the foundation of my thought process for more than 20 years. I hope to do that for you with this book.

Michael Boyle

INTRODUCTION

Strength and Conditioning Coaching is a "how to" book. It moves from the task of equipping a weightroom, through a discussion of programming concepts, and eventually to actual workouts with detailed explanations. My philosophy has always been based on the belief that athletes aren't limited by genetics. Speed, movement ability, strength and power are all qualities that can and should be improved. This is a basic primer on how to make those improvements, how to get things done and the reasons we do them.

The concepts are meant to be both simple and also utilitarian:

What equipment do I need?

How many plates do I need?

How much space do I need?

How many sets and reps should I have my athletes do?

What exercises work best?

The information in this book is just one man's opinion. However, that opinion is based on 40 years of working in facilities that weren't perfect, often with small or nonexistent budgets. The advice you'll read might be the most efficient and effective way to do things, but it won't be the only way.

This book is ideal for the high school or small college coach who has to deal with the realities of time, space and money. While reading it, put aside preconceived notions about the process of strength and conditioning. Instead, think about practicing the art of common sense.

"Common sense is not very common."
~ Voltaire

While you read, keep your mind open.

"Don't believe everything you read, and don't read only what you believe."
~ Martin Rooney

We often discount good ideas because of their simplicity. As coaches and personal trainers, we continue to jump on and off the latest bandwagons, but I encourage you to stay with ideas that work and be wary of anything that seems too good to be true.

Great strength and conditioning coaches constantly scrutinize their programs. Every week, there's something that makes me think about changing our programs. These aren't knee-jerk reactions but rather are the acceptance and appreciation of the many strength coaches, sport coaches and physical therapists pushing the envelope and developing better techniques.

At Mike Boyle Strength and Conditioning, we don't copy the programs of successful groups, teams or athletes. Instead, we evaluate each technique or concept for inclusion in our programs. Many coaches attempt to duplicate or replicate the programs of the most successful teams, but much of a program's success may be due to recruiting, coaching, genetics or even drugs.

Seek out the techniques of those who consistently produce great results in less-than-great situations instead of copying successful teams or coaches.

Assessing Credibility in the Internet Age

Don't copy the routines of internet coaches. Seriously, don't. Real coaches make the mistake of following internet "coaches" who don't actually coach anyone. It's unfortunate that people can become experts based on some lies, some half-truths and a laptop, but that's our current reality.

Years ago, Tim Edgerton, a UK strength and conditioning coach, named me the most influential man in strength and conditioning. I was initially flattered, but my excitement waned when I saw the rest of the list. Tim's list of "influencers" was about 50-percent non-coaches. Many were academic NSCA types, plus a few internet marketers and a few coaches.

There's a constant flow of X/Twitter articles and posts from non-coaches or at least non-active coaches. The internet is riddled with people who've never done our jobs telling us how to do our jobs.

It seems to be the same people (usually guys) writing redundant articles. These are often about what we're doing wrong in the team sports world and are usually long and drawn out without much actual information.

Additionally, the writers seem to have the same resume. "_____ *is one of the world's most sought-after experts in the field of strength and conditioning and…"*

The next time you read one of these resumes, google the author and then ask yourself these few simple questions:

Is the writer one of the world's most sought-after experts in any area?

Does the writer make a living coaching, or does he or she make a living by writing? In Alwyn Cosgrove's words, "Have they been there, done that and are they still doing it?"

Has the writer made a consistent living actually coaching or training people?

What does the writer do every day? Does this person sit at a computer and write articles or work in the field?

Did the writer help anyone get better?

Is the resume legitimate or are the qualifications and client list inflated?

Do a little research and find out. Make sure the article you're studying was written by a person who's been successful doing the work. You might be surprised at what you learn—let's not bankroll some guy who just read *The 4-Hour Workweek.*

Don't copy workouts designed by people using performance-enhancing drugs written for people using performance-enhancing drugs. Performance-enhancing drugs allow tolerance of higher loads, higher volumes and more frequent training. These people often get better in spite of a program, not because of it.

More is not better, particularly in the drug-tested sports world. We now strive for the *minimum effective dose.* This is the least amount of work that produces the desired result. Most young athletes and many young coaches feel that if two sets are good, four sets are obviously better. In truth, they may be overtaxing themselves and their athletes and disrupting the recuperative process.

When thinking of a strength program, try to remember strength training is a simple game of stimulus and response. Training is just a stimulus; the gains are made in the recuperative period. The response occurs *after* the workout and is affected by the quality and quantity of the workouts and the quality of the recovery. Rest and nutrition have as much to do with success as does the program. In other words, "Don't let today's workout ruin tomorrow's." I'll give Tony Holler credit for that one.

The real key to a successful strength and conditioning program is injury reduction. The old coaches' joke is that the most desirable ability in a player is *avail-*ability. I've used the term "injury prevention" in the past, but only divine intervention can actually prevent injury. Injury *reduction* is a better goal.

Semantics aside, statistics don't lie. If your injuries decrease and your wins increase, you're successful. Wins can be affected by talent and coaching, but in general, injury trends won't be as affected by these factors. Your number one goal is injury reduction—performance enhancement is the secondary goal.

I noticed an interesting trend during my 30 years of college coaching. As our program evolved from a traditional powerlifting and Olympic lifting program to a more functionally based program, our strength numbers stayed consistent, but our injury incidence decreased drastically.

Filling Buckets?

There's a kid's book my son read in the first grade called *Have You Filled a Bucket Today*? To summarize, bucket fillers provide the good stuff and help fill your bucket. Bucket dippers dip in your bucket and make you feel bad. I fell in love with the simple analogy of being a bucket filler.

When I discuss training, I find myself using what we call "the bucket analogy." My advice is always simple: I tell coaches to fill the empty buckets. Don't fill a bucket that's full.

If we look at each quality—strength, power, endurance, conditioning—as a bucket to be filled, the answer of the "what to do" question becomes simple: Be bucket fillers. Fill the empty buckets; don't overflow full buckets.

If the strength bucket is empty, fill it. If the muscle endurance bucket is already full, leave it alone. Don't worry or complain about who filled it or how, just move to the next bucket.

When I say to "fill the bucket," I don't mean to fill it to the absolute brim. We know what happens when we try to do that—it overflows as soon as someone tries to pick it up or move it. Instead, leave a little room at the top to give yourself a small buffer to avoid spillage. In our world, it's better to leave a bit of room in the bucket than overdo it and run our athletes in to the ground. We want them to get stronger, but when we get greedy, we overflow their recovery capacity and create a mess.

Remember, any fool can make an athlete tired… and many do.

Thoughts for Young Coaches

When people ask what I'd tell a young coach just starting out, I start by reminding them there might be a reason they have two eyes, two ears and only one mouth. Coaches should strive to watch and listen at least twice as much as they talk. And to that, let's add the proven fact that young people drastically overestimate how much they know. Google "the Dunning-Kruger effect."

I'd also remind them to listen to music and to the words of the songs. One of my favorites is a James Taylor tune called *Lonesome Road*. Here's my favorite lyric from the song:

"If I'd stopped to listen once or twice, if I closed my mouth and opened my eyes, I'd not be on this road tonight."

I'd tell them to read. A young coach should have a self-improvement plan that extends beyond personal appearance…and into the real world. And please don't say you don't like to read. If you struggle to read, listen to audiobooks.

The clichés about reading and readers are endless. Readers are leaders.

"I have known no wise people who didn't read all the time, none, zero."
~ Charlie Munger

If you're asking yourself who Charlie Munger is, you need to read more.

Looking the part of a coach is fine, but new coaches need to understand what "looking the part" actually means. Coaches aren't auditioning for the role of a refrigerator. Modern strength and conditioning coaches need to be athletes.

If you're muscular, the world will know. You don't need to wear your little brother or sister's clothes to show the world your fitness. You also don't need to post partially nude photos of yourself or pictures of yourself lifting. No one cares how much you can lift. Please don't post videos of your PRs.

When I look at resumes and I see bodybuilding, powerlifting or Olympic lifting listed under hobbies, I'm not impressed. When I see team sports participation such as track and field, that's when my eyes light up.

Acting the part is more important than looking the part. Be professional; decline if the new football coach needs a clown to assume the role of sideline court jester. Want to be a hype man? Maybe consider cheerleading from the outset.

My Road to the "Top"

I've been lifting weights since around 1973. I started in the basement with a 110-pound York set and a wall chart. My father was a high school teacher, coach and Hall of Fame football player in college, and I planned to be just like him.

My football career was ended by two serious problems that afflict far too many athletes—lack of size and talent were two things I couldn't overcome. While trying to conquer my limitations, I discovered I had some fast-twitch muscle fibers and I liked lifting weights.

Lifting kept me sane after giving up football. I pursued athletic training and dabbled in powerlifting in college.

In true Malcolm Gladwell *Outliers* fashion, during my first two years in college I had a dorm director named Mike Woicek. What luck! Mike was the former Dallas Cowboys and New England Patriots strength and conditioning coach; at one time he was tied with a Patriots quarterback for the most Super Bowl rings in the history of the NFL (6). Rusty Jones, former Indianapolis Colts and Buffalo Bills strength and conditioning coach, was also at Springfield College at that time. From the beginning, I had great mentors and role models.

I left Springfield College after five years with a master's degree and took a job at Boston University as an assistant athletic trainer. I wanted to be a strength coach. It was 1982 and I was about 185 pounds soaking wet. I didn't look like a strength coach then and still don't.

But I took the plunge after just six months—I quit my fulltime job as an athletic trainer and became the volunteer strength coach—I began my journey by giving up a salary and benefits in favor of a volunteer job. Very few schools even had fulltime strength and conditioning coaches at the time. I tended bar at night to pay the bills and threw myself into my exciting new unpaid job.

My initial work was with our basketball team. Rick Pitino, the coach, soon left for greener pastures and former NBA player and future NBA coach John Kuester took over and asked me to run a preseason program. I was then able to convince former Harvard football coaching legend Tim Murphy, who at that time was the Boston University offensive line coach, to let me run the off-season football program.

At the time, I was a former football player, a basketball coach's son and a former competitive powerlifter, but I became a "hockey expert" at the urging of the hockey coaches at Boston University. Boston U is to college hockey what Notre Dame or USC are to college football. I began to analyze hockey and quickly discovered no one in Boston was training professional hockey players. I'd found my niche.

I met a hockey agent named Bob Murray and talked him into sending me a few minor league clients—I told him no professional athletes. I needed desperate people who'd listen to a football guy tell them how to make it to the NHL. I also started training high school hockey players because I needed the money. That may have been the smartest thing I've ever done.

When some of my new minor league clients made the NHL, the Boston Bruins offered me a part-time job as their strength and conditioning coach. With a little money from BU and some from the Bruins, I gave up the bar business and was now a fulltime strength and conditioning coach with two jobs.

I worked from 8:30 AM to 11:30 AM with the Bruins and then drove to BU and opened the weightroom at noon. I coached every day at BU from 12:00 to 7:00 PM, with some additional 6:00 AM football activity before Bruins practice during the winter. I'd either go to a BU game or go back to the old Boston Garden at 7:00 PM to train injured players or those who didn't dress out for the game... and would try to coerce a few players to work out after the game. I'd get home about 11:00 PM, not a bad day for an eight-month season.

My speaking career began at roughly the same time. Those "speaking engagements" were to middle school hockey players in groups of maybe a dozen at hockey camps, but they were paid jobs that allowed me to get comfortable in front of a tougher audience.

Then Chris Poirier and Perform Better® gave me a big break when they began their Perform Better clinics. I was one of the first speakers and, as with any good job, I never left.

I did those two jobs for 10 seasons and then found time to leave my fulltime job at BU to open Mike Boyle Strength and Conditioning. We were one of the first for-profit centers in the country. As Alwyn Cosgrove and Jason Ferrugia so aptly described in their article, "The Business," I was rapidly becoming an overnight success one 12-hour day at a time.

The rest is simple: I kept doing what I was doing.

I worked on my business. I put in my 10,000 hours. I coached athletes and I coached coaches. I took chances and was willing to work long hours.

It wasn't easy. Except for my six-month athletic training job at BU, I didn't have a fulltime job with health insurance until I was 30 years old.

Most people give up just before their big break arrives. Don't let that be you. Your big break may be right around the corner. Keep moving forward.

It's Not the Program; It's the Coaching

Why does an assistant coach go to a new position, institute the same program used in the former job, yet fail to get similar results? Or why are the results not the same when a head strength coach moves on and the assistant takes over? The obvious answer is talent, but that's an oversimplification.

It's usually not the program; it's the coach. In the football world, legendary coach Bum Phillips described Paul Bear Bryant's coaching this way:

"He can take his'n and beat your'n and take your'n and beat his'n."

In other words, if you and Bryant switched rosters, the following year he'd beat you with your former team.

A great strength coach with a mediocre program is much better than a great strength program and a mediocre coach. A program is a piece of paper or a file on a laptop. Programs don't motivate athletes or create accountability. That paper can't figure out what's inside a person and discover how to access it. A great coach can do all those things.

Great coaches teach, motivate and create an accountability system. They'll figure out what makes each person tick and use that knowledge to get results.

All of our programs at MBSC are the same. Our philosophy never changes. Want to get fast? Run sprints. Want to get strong? Lift weights. The difference is in the selling, both to athletes and coaches. The other difference is in knowing what makes each athlete tick.

Another legendary coach, the late quarterback guru Tom Martinez, described it this way in *Outliers*:

"Every kid's life is a mix of shit and ice cream. If the kid has had too much shit, I mix in some ice cream. If he has had too much ice cream, I mix in some shit."

Martinez knew there's a different key to every lock. To paraphrase Dan John, the key is to find the key.

There's a reason strength and conditioning coaches like Mike Woicek, Al Miller, Rusty Jones and Johnny Parker had teams in almost every Super Bowl over a 15-year period. They're great coaches who get the best out of their players.

There's also a reason a coach like Phil Jackson succeeded in circumstances as different as Chicago and LA: Coaching matters.

Coaches change lives. Programs don't. The people will always matter more than the paper.

Become a Great Coach

If you want to succeed at anything, including coaching, you must become a good person. People often miss the boat when looking for success. Success is simple. It's not about how many letters you have after your name or the appearance of your muscles.

Instead, work hard and be nice. Remember:

"No one cares how much you know, until they know how much you care."
~ Theodore Roosevelt

Great coaches have a service mentality. Their coaching isn't all about them. In fact, it's rarely about them. You can usually identify a great coach right away. They greet you, smile and shake your hand. They treat you as an equal and as a guest in their facility.

It's much easier to impart knowledge than it is to try to change personal qualities. I can make our coaches and trainers smarter, but I can't make them nicer. Believe me, I've tried.

Internship

The internship route is the best way for us to find great coaches. These are like tryouts—interns don't expect to be hired. We simply keep the ones we like. It's perfect. Most of our staff was "hired" this way. Those who fail the work ethic and "nice person" tests simply move on.

During your internships, pay attention to the interns' work ethics. Do the potential employees arrive early? Do they stay late? When you ask for volunteers, are they first in line? Or do they frequently ask for time off? Are they often sick? Do they have multiple family emergencies during a short internship? These are all signs of a poor work ethic. Certainly, things come up, but when you're 21, life shouldn't get in the way too much.

Nice person tests are simple. Watch people. How do your interns interact with their peers? With athletes and clients? With delivery and service people? You want people who are nice to everyone, all the time. You want people who care about other people. These are who we should teach and help succeed.

We have our interns read Dale Carnegie's *How to Win Friends and Influence People*. This self-help classic is step one to becoming a great coach. Add a little Steven Covey and some John Maxwell, and they're well on their way.

Interviews

Do interviews work if you don't have the luxury of having interns? Hiring through interviews is tough;

it's hard to learn much about a person's temperament from a resume and a half-hour conversation.

If you must go that route, check the applicant's references before the interview. The best reference is from someone you know and trust, and the worst is from a current boss. A current boss might lie to get rid of a bad employee. However, you can ask something like, "What will I say to you next time we speak?" This often elicits the truth. The thought of a callback a few weeks after a hire is unnerving to someone who's lying. What was originally a great reference will sometimes turn lukewarm.

After references, consider first impressions. I only hire people who truly want to work at Mike Boyle Strength and Conditioning. If they ask too many questions about benefits and time off, we won't get along too well. I need people who are excited to come to work and help people every day.

How are they dressed for the interview? I still love seeing a tie, even though I don't own one. A little old-school respect goes a long way at our facility. It may be an interview for a job in a gym, but it's still a job interview. We've had people show up in sweatpants and untied shoes. No thanks.

In our facility, I want to see people who've worked at networking. Ideally, they've already visited us, taken a tour and met some of the staff. If they live near Boston and have never been in our facility, why would I want to hire them?

Becoming a great coach is more about upbringing than anything else. Work to find the right people. If you look for certifications, degrees and prior experience, you're missing the boat. Instead, look at personality and work ethic. Knowledge is easy to obtain, but personality and work habits are tough to instill after the hire.

Hire great coaches; they'll make you look smart and will help create a successful business and a winning team.

Now that we've considered or built a quality staff, let's talk about how to set things up to build a successful business. We'll design the facility in the first chapter.

CHAPTER 1
DESIGNING AND EQUIPPING YOUR FACILITY

Equipping a facility is our first issue. Avoiding mistakes at this point will determine how well you'll be able to design and implement a program as you progress. Great programming ideas are only ideas if poor logistics in the facility prevent your concepts from being turned into quality programs. Mistakes in choosing equipment are expensive to undo.

Beer and Chocolate Chip Ice Cream

To properly equip a facility, you'll need to consider both equipment usage and the traffic flow of the facility. As you design the space usage, it's crucial to remember that the design isn't about what you like.

Let's use the beer and chocolate chip ice cream example. Beer and ice cream are two of my favorite nutritional choices, but when people ask me for nutrition advice, I don't recommend beer and ice cream because good nutrition choices aren't about what I like. As you start to design your facility, ask yourself if you're making a good decision or a "beer and chocolate ice cream" choice.

Traffic Flow

In designing your space, envision your traffic plan. Where do people enter? Where do they roll and stretch? Where do they warm up? Where do they do plyos?

Flow is everything in a facility. If you're a high school or a college strength coach, the flow of the floor determines how many kids you can serve. If you're in the private sector, flow determines how much money you can make.

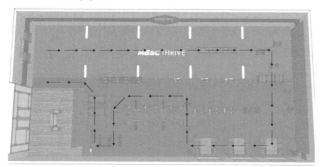

Figure 1.1—Designing a weightroom for traffic flow

Turf and Sprint Space

In the first edition of this facilities book, I didn't discuss the idea of adding turf space to a weightroom. In 1997, I designed a new facility at Boston University, where we put in four lanes of rubber track surface for sprints, jumps and active general warm-ups. Every person who walked in the room at that time said things like, "What kind of equipment is going here?" or "Didn't all the equipment arrive yet?"

In 1997, people weren't used to seeing empty space in a weightroom, but now it's common. Back then, I regularly had to tell people we were leaving open space for sprints and plyometrics. Most coaches had never entertained the idea of having open space in a weightroom. Sadly, some still don't.

In current facilities, open space for sprints, jumps and sled work is standard, but not long ago, this type of space in a strength and conditioning facility was a progressive idea. I now suggest at least 50/50 open space versus space devoted to equipment.

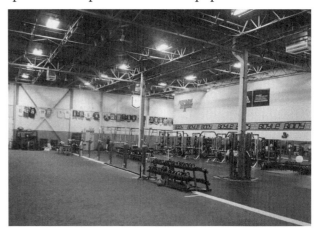

Figure 1.2—Open space is key!
The longer the "sprint lane," the better.

I recommend turf over a rubber surface. Turf not only looks cool, but is a far better surface for sprinting, jumping, direction change and sled work.

Sprint Space

In training athletes, sprint space is now my top consideration. Can the athletes run at least a 10-yard or 10-meter sprint and have space to decelerate? In fact, if I were designing a facility today, I'd pad the end wall so people could decelerate into it. Sprint training is the velocity-based training of the future. Allocate space for sprints and sled sprints.

I spoke with one of my former assistants who'd just finished a new room and he said, "We don't have room to sprint." My response was, "Take some stuff out." Yes, it's that important.

Designing the "Weight" Section of the Weightroom

Some type of multi-use rack system yields the greatest weightroom usage per square foot. There's never enough space. With the emphasis on functional training, space has become more important than equipment. This means equipment in our current computer-dominated-language must "multitask." This points to the combination of some type of power rack.

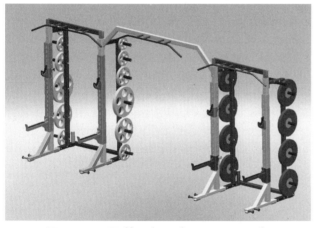

Figure 1.3—Half-racks with connectors is the number-one design key.

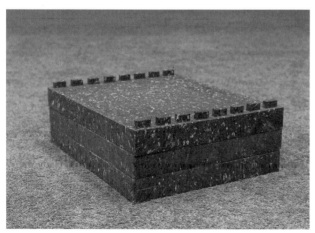

Figure 1.4—Clean blocks make hang cleans simple to implement.

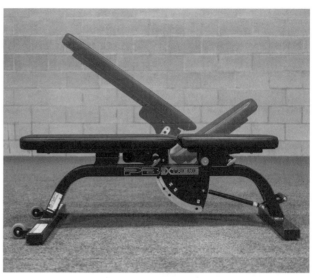

Figure 1.5—Always buy adjustable benches. You can always keep the bench flat, but a flat bench won't incline.

An adjustable flat-to-incline bench and a set of Olympic lifting blocks allow athletes to perform almost any exercise in a small area and make for great usage of each valuable square foot.

Figure 1.6 below clearly shows how utilitarian a weightroom can be when properly designed. A room designed around a good rack system is designed for team or group usage.

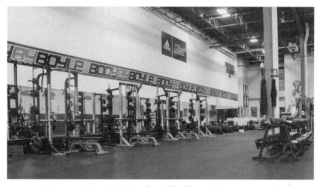

Figure 1.6—Racks, dumbbells and open space!

Choosing Racks

I'm well known for changing my mind and admitting when I'm wrong. In the first edition of this book I wrote:

"Don't buy the currently popular half-racks. Half-racks have become increasingly popular over the past five years, but the truth is a half-rack is actually a half of a power rack that doesn't cost half as much, but is in fact half as useful. Half-racks are designed with pull-up bars, but the reality is that you can't simultaneously use the rack for squats and pull-ups

because the squat bar is in the way...Half-racks look good, but function poorly."

However, you'll see we've gone to all half-racks if you visit either of the Mike Boyle Strength and Conditioning locations. What made me change my mind? The new Perform Better rack system eliminated the big drawback of the half-rack.

I've always liked the look of a half-rack. It makes the room appear less cluttered. It wasn't until I ordered six of them in 2004 and realized we couldn't do chins and squats together that the drawback became obvious.

The Perform Better racks with connectors take a design flaw and turn it into a strength. A minimum of six feet between racks is necessary. Many people used that space to place a tree for plate storage. As rack systems evolved, most racks come with plate storage built in. The between-rack space became dead space because we still needed at least three feet between bar ends for safety, meaning the racks themselves still must be at least six feet apart.

The rack itself is about four feet wide, but the bar is seven feet long. This means 18 inches of the bar is outside the rack on either end. With three feet between bar ends, there are six feet between racks.

The idea of connectors between the racks takes dead space in the weightroom and makes it useable. The between-rack space gets used efficiently whether you're doing chin-ups or mounting some type of suspension trainer. If you like to pair exercises, this is a huge bonus.

If you read the first edition of this book and decided against half-racks, you might want to look at the new Perform Better racks and reconsider.

The facilities we currently design are in stark contrast to the weightrooms of the 1980s and '90s that were designed in "Noah's Ark" style. The coach simply ordered two of everything in the Noah's Ark weightroom. The rooms often resembled a Gold's Gym more than a strength and conditioning facility.

These facilities weren't at all conducive to team or group training. In fact, a facility designed with too much machinery actually causes bottlenecks as athletes wait for a piece of equipment that's in short supply. With a good rack and a large supply of dumbbells, athletes never wait for equipment.

Inlaid Platforms

Our first facilities were sold on the value of platforms for Olympic lifting, although I'm not sure why. It was another one of those things we did because everyone else did it. In reality, platforms are like placeholders that say, "Don't step here; you might get a weight dropped on you."

We now use inlaid platforms instead of raised platforms. The "platforms" are flooring made to look like a platform. Although serving the same purpose, they eliminate a large cost and tripping hazard.

Cleaning up also becomes much easier. Raised platforms created great areas to accumulate dust.

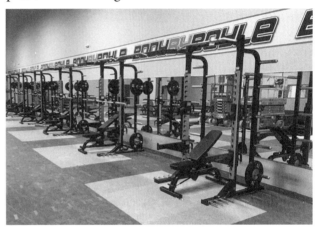

Figure 1.7—Inlaid platforms designate space with no trip hazard.

Essential Equipment List

The following is a sample equipment list that includes the necessary items for a moderate-budget facility. These items should be included in your plan for one simple reason: If you're in a school setting, you may not get a second chance.

Purchasing is a funny thing—and you seem to get one large shot. You don't score any extra points for coming in under budget in university settings. The only thing coming in under budget ever gets you is a smaller future budget. Spend every cent. In fact, go over budget. Be a little extravagant. It will give you room to work if they ask you to cut the proposed budget.

The list shown on the following page is based on four power racks and four Olympic lift areas with inlaid platforms. This is by no means an all-inclusive list, but it is a good starting point.

4 power racks with connectors
4 adjustable benches
4 power bars (bars designed for squats, bench press, etc.)
4 Olympic bars (order bars suitable for Olympic lifts)
4 sets of clean blocks
16 45-pound plates (4 per bar)
16 45-pound bumper plates (4 per bar)
8 25-pound plates (2 per bar)
8 25-pound bumper plates (2 per bar)
32 10-pound plates (4 per bar)
16 5-pound plates (2 per bar)
16 2.5-pound plates (2 per bar)
16 1.25-pound plates (2 per bar)
4 sets of Powerblocks (85-pound set or the monster 125s)
4 pulley systems (Keiser Infinity Trainer or Ancore Rack Mounted)
4 slide boards (10-foot Ultraslide)
4 mini slide boards
4 landmine attachments
4 foam plyo box sets (12", 18", 24", 30")
12 Stroops Yellow Safety toner loops
12 Soft Toss med balls (4–4 pound, 4–6 pound, 4–8 pound)
4 sets of mini hurdles 6", 12", 18", 24" (6 of each)
16 Rollga foam rollers
4 sprint sleds with pro waist cinch belts
4 drive sleds

Facility Design Guidelines

Bill Kroll, the former University of Illinois strength and conditioning coach, wrote an excellent series of articles on facility design for the *NSCA Journal* in the 1980s and early 1990s. The concepts Kroll advocated have dictated how I designed and redesigned weightrooms for the last 10 years.

Kroll also advocated the use of power rack systems. He gave very specific guidelines for design of the room.

Allow 100 square feet of space per person.

If you have a team of 25 players you'd like to train at the same time, you'll need a minimum of 2,500 square feet. This is a minimum for a facility using the connected power racks concept and having minimal machines or cardiovascular pieces.

Single-use machines and cardio pieces generally take up big footprints, but can only accommodate one athlete. This is the biggest mistake people make in planning a facility.

One hundred square feet accounts for people plus essential equipment. Architects often say the room size allotted for a new project like this is too large, but they aren't thinking about the combination of people plus equipment.

This is a common mistake made in many arena weightrooms when architects are involved. I've frequently seen professional sports teams with tiny facilities in brand-new arenas. Use 100 square feet per team member as a bare minimum. Use a larger number like 200 square feet if you plan on having a volume of single-station equipment or an array of cardio pieces.

If you'd like a large open space for warm-up or post-workout stretching, budget for this also. You'll never get a second chance to add more space unless you move to a new facility. Get as much space as possible, and don't worry about equipping it. The old facility philosophy was to set up a health club-like environment. That's the Noah's Ark weightroom.

If you intend to train groups or teams, having one or two of any piece of equipment only creates problems and bottlenecks the facility. Pieces like large glute-ham benches and reverse hypers become seldom-used space stealers. You need to have at least four of something to use it in a team program; otherwise, you create funnels.

If you're going to order four of any piece, make sure it isn't a single-use piece. That's what makes the connected rack idea so attractive. You should have as many of these rack set-ups as you can fit and very little else, particularly when on a tight budget or tight for space.

Get as much ceiling height as possible.

Specify at least 12 feet from floor to ceiling. Ten feet is the bare minimum for six-foot athletes to perform overhead lifts. You have to factor in athlete height, arm length, platform height if you intend to use raised platforms instead of inlaid and the diameter of a 20-kilogram or 45-pound plate. Architects just won't think of these factors.

BE SPECIFIC. When we built our hockey strength facility at Boston University in 2004, parts of the room were 8′6.″ We had athletes who could jump and hit their heads on the ceiling and had to relocate some mechanicals to provide enough overhead room in certain areas so they could lift bars overhead. The rationale I was given for the low ceiling was that I stated the ceiling height should be *"12 feet high or as high as possible."* I was told I should have specified a *minimum* of 12 feet. The architects deemed 8′6″ to be "as high as possible" based on the need to run a large piece of metal ductwork through the room. Be specific!

On another note, a facility with a lot of ceiling height is more aesthetically pleasing.

Put the mirrors 24 inches off the floor.

If you do this, no one will ever lean a plate on the wall and break a mirror. Athletes aren't supposed to lean plates against the wall, but they always do—and low or floor-to-ceiling mirrors often get broken.

Demand bright light.

In our 2004 facility build-out, I was specific with the architect about lighting. I wanted the room to be daylight bright. The architect told me not to worry, that it was under control. The primary result was a low ceiling and darkness. The secondary result was an almost $200,000 estimate to improve the lighting quality.

Don't let your architect fur out your walls.

Architects often want to cover a block or poured concrete wall with sheetrock for aesthetic reasons. Don't let them. You can never have enough concrete or block walls to throw against in medicine ball training. Throwing a med ball with a partner doesn't compare to throwing against a wall. In our case, the contractors had to tear out studs and drywall that covered a poured concrete wall that I specified was to be left uncovered. I was told it was done for aesthetics. We had it removed.

Consider a "built in" medicine ball wall. Our newest MBSC facility is in an all-metal building, and we built a 20 x 10-foot concrete block medicine ball wall. And I wish we'd gone 40 feet in length.

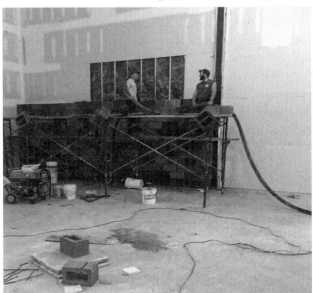

Figure 1.8—A medicine ball wall is essential. Make one if you have to.

Allot 10 feet per Olympic bar.

People always counter my bar space suggestion with statements like, "An Olympic bar is only seven feet long," but they aren't thinking about having space between bars to load and unload plates. Allotting 10 feet per bar means each bar will have a three-foot space between the ends. This way there won't be accidents loading and unloading bars.

You'll need 40 feet of uninterrupted wall space for four normal racks. The connected power rack idea will take up slightly more linear space, but the fact that you're gaining space for chin-ups and suspension trainers makes the trade-off worth it. The only exception is that you can have one-and-a-half feet at the beginning or end of any row of racks and still have a safe environment.

1.5'	7'	3'	7'	3'	7'	3'	7'	1.5'
	BAR		BAR		BAR		BAR	

This setup indicates how a four-rack layout would work along a 40-foot wall. One-and-a-half feet is fine at either end of a run, but three feet is essential between bars.

Equipment Guidelines

Don't buy 35-pound plates.

This is a simple money-saver. Thirty-fives take up rack space, make your racks unorganized and provide no benefit. You only need 25s and 10s. Save your money; don't buy 35s.

Get twice as many 10-pound plates as 25s, 5s and 2.5s.

Many weight combinations will require two 10-pound plates on each end of the bar. This is never the case with 25-pound plates, 5-pound plates or 2.5-pound plates. Two 10s make a 20, not a 25. You need twice as many 10s as 25s, 5s or 2.5s.

Get dumbbells in 2.5-pound increments or PowerBlock dumbbells.

Dumbbells are normally sold in 5-pound increments. This is standard. However, more companies now manufacture dumbbells in 2.5-pound increments. This is a big deal because 5-pound increments don't allow younger or less-trained athletes to progress at reasonable rates. For example, when less-experienced athletes advance from two 15-pound dumbbells to two 20-pound dumbbells, they're progressing from 30 pounds to 40 pounds, an increase of 33 percent. I hope you wouldn't ask a stronger athlete to go from 60-pound dumbbells to 80-pound dumbbells in one week.

For anyone contemplating outfitting a home gym, check out the PowerBlock and SportBlock systems. Every set has the capacity to provide an interchangeable weight with the adjustable dumbbell system.

Get 15-, 25-, and 35-pound Olympic bars.

Many young or female athletes have little or no strength training background and may need lighter bars in the beginning. Most equipment companies now stock these new lighter bars.

Younger athletes should look like everyone else in the weightroom. In the psychology of a strength training facility, younger or weaker athletes are often intimidated just being in the facility. Providing them with equipment that allows them to fit in drastically increases enjoyment and compliance.

Over the past year, we've found less need for the 15- and 25-pound bars and now use 35s more. In a new facility, I'd buy one 15-pound bar and one 25-pound bar, but most young athletes easily handle the 35-pound bar in things like the hang clean or bench press.

Get 1.25-pound Olympic plates.

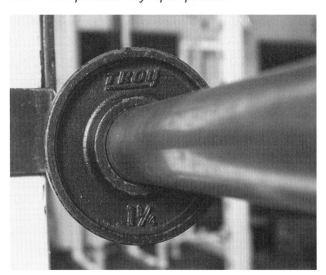

Figure 1.9—1.25 plates are a key to progressive resistance.

You can purchase 1.25-pound Olympic plates, although they're not found in most gyms. The same logic described earlier in reference to 2.5-increment dumbbells applies here. Moving from 45 to 50 pounds is only a 5-pound jump, but it's also a 10-percent jump. Many female athletes won't be able to make this type of progression. The male example again illustrates this point: Ask a male athlete to jump from 300 to 330 in the bench press in one week. This is only a 10-percent jump but would be impossible for any athlete.

Design your facility with success in mind. The key to designing and equipping a facility is to think first about who you're going to train. How many people will use the facility and at what times? You need to look at age, gender and level of experience.

When designing, think about multi-purpose and user-friendly equipment with plenty of space. Those are the keys. Success isn't about fancy equipment but about facility function. Envision your facility as a factory to produce strength, speed and power to create a smooth-running assembly line.

Weightroom Rules

We're all about creating the right training environment. To do that, we need rules. Athletes may view the rules as restrictive, but there's a method to the madness. The following are the weightroom rules I've developed over the years. We've used these rules at both Boston University and Mike Boyle Strength and Conditioning.

Rule 1: Treat people the way you want to be treated. They call this the "Golden Rule" for a reason. You already know this.

Rule 2: No lifting gloves. I dislike all weightroom paraphernalia. Gloves, long pants, work boots and flannel shirts have no place in the weightroom. I dislike gloves because I dislike guys who don't want calluses. Workers have callused hands. I want workers. My upperclassmen loved it when a new guy showed up with gloves. They let the poor kid come into the weightroom with gloves on just to see me tell him to put them back in his locker.

Rule 3: No personal headphones, earbuds, etc. We want interaction in the weightroom, not everybody jamming to their own tunes. Earbuds, Airpods and similar devices are unsafe. Some guy blaring Drake may not hear you when you say, "Look out. I just dropped a really heavy dumbbell."

Rule 4: No music that contains obscenities or racial or sexual references. I didn't want to hear certain words, but I had trouble figuring out how to make this point clear. I felt like the late George Carlin with the *Seven Dirty Words You Can't Say on TV*. I came up with this: No derogatory racial terms and no reference to sex with family members. I tell my athletes, "You want rap or hip hop, download the clean version at iTunes or get me Walmart rap."

Rule 5: No tank tops for men. This is an incredibly sexist rule. Women can wear tank tops, but men can't. I know this is a double standard. However, men in tank tops spend too much time looking at themselves in the mirror. Additionally, if you allow men to wear tank tops, they'll continue to cut them down until there is barely any shirt left. For women, tank tops are all about empowerment and confidence. There are far too many negative messages about body image in their lives. This isn't the case with men; hence, the rationale for my double standard.

Rule 5A: Wear a shirt! I can't believe how many X/Twitter videos I see of male high school and college athletes lifting shirtless. First, there are sanitary issues. Secondly, it looks incredibly unprofessional.

Rule 6: Shorts must cover both ends of your butt. This is a unisex rule, but applies differently. I think it's great that a young woman feels good about her body; however, I don't want a peek at her underwear every time she bends over. Exercises like hip lifts and single-leg straight-leg deadlifts become too adventurous in these cases. The opposite is true for men. For a young woman, we're covering cheeks; for a young man, we're avoiding the jail look. This is simply my old-fashioned coach persona at work. Pull up your shorts and cover your underwear. The truth is, you look like an idiot with your hat on sideways and your underwear showing.

Rule 7: Don't be an ___hole. If you want to yell, scream and throw weights, go somewhere else. The big impression is made in lifting the weights, not in putting them down. If you lift heavy weights, people will notice.

CHAPTER 2
BUILDING A STRONG PROGRAM FOUNDATION

A strong foundation isn't only the key to building a home, but a successful strength and conditioning program as well. The old adage about not building a house on sand couldn't be more true. A good strength and conditioning program, like a good house, needs a strong foundation.

However, the converse can also be true. The foundation should be the underpinnings on which a program is based, but the foundation shouldn't completely determine the function of the house. We still want modern kitchens and baths and wireless internet to go with our strong foundation.

What does all this have to do with strength and conditioning? Too many coaches never build past the foundation. Olympic lifting and powerlifting are excellent systems that teach a strong technical background and emphasize multi-joint lifts. However, much like the invention of modern plumbing and the internet, strength and conditioning is constantly advancing. To be successful, we need to advance with it.

Function, speed, power and core training are only a few of the examples of advances that should be incorporated into a sound program. There are far too many ostriches in our profession, content to coach with their heads in the sand.

I trace my foundation back through Al Vermeil (eight World Championships) and Mike Woicek (six Super Bowl wins) to the late Ken Leistner (*The Steel Tip*) and Bill Starr (*The Strong Shall Survive*). I've listened to and read the works of all these men and have never moved too far from the basic concepts they taught. However, I've also incorporated the work of great minds in rehab like Gray Cook and Stuart McGill.

The most frightening person in the world is the one who believes he or she has all the answers. I spend countless hours reading and listening to people in the fields of strength and conditioning, rehab, psychology and business. The more research I do, the more I realize how little I know.

Coaches frequently try to do too much too soon when starting a strength and conditioning program. The key to developing a successful program is to decide what you want your athletes to learn, and then focus on one major lift per day.

At clinics, I speak with coaches interested in starting or improving the strength and conditioning program at their schools. They're looking for guidance in setting up a program and almost always want to talk sets and reps. Coaches ask, "Should I do Westside?" "Should I use the TriPhasic?" Instead, I want to discuss organization and administrative concepts because these are the real keys to a successful program. Setup and execution make the program run, not sets and reps.

A bad program done well is better than a good program done poorly.

A bad program done with consistency and effort will be more beneficial than a great program done inconsistently and with little effort.

Keep it simple. If you're a one-person show, consider adhering to the following guidelines.

Make sure all your athletes are on board.

If you're starting a high school or a collegiate program, forget uncooperative seniors. Dealing with seniors who "already know how to lift" is the major source of frustration in starting a high school or college program. Separate these athletes right away. If they don't cooperate, get rid of them— they'll be gone soon anyway.

If you're coaching alone, consider using only one coaching-intensive lift per day.

Exercises like goblet squats, trap bar deadlifts or the Olympic movements are considered coaching-intensive. Coaches must watch every set to help engrain the correct motor pattern into their athletes. If different athletes are doing goblet squats and hang cleans at the same time, which do you watch, the hang cleans or the goblet squats?

29

Don't force yourself to make this decision.

For example, have them do split squats instead of goblet squats on the day they do hang cleans, and do push-ups instead of bench press on the day they goblet squat. On goblet squat day, consider not doing an Olympic movement. Instead, perform some type of squat jump or trap bar jump as the explosive exercise. This process of doing one coaching intensive lift per day may only last a year, but it ensures your athletes won't be practicing poor patterns without supervision.

Get all your administrative work done prior to the start of sessions.

Coaches sitting at a laptop or getting stuck in the office instead of coaching is the biggest failure in strength and conditioning today. If you need workouts created on a laptop, prep them during non-training time. The job is strength and conditioning *coach*. Many coaches get caught up in having great programs on paper, and ultimately end up with lousy lifters. Let the paperwork wait so you can get into the coaching.

Coach.

Coach like this is your sport.

Many coaches ask, "Can you give me a program?" I always give the same answer, "I could, but it probably won't work." Some programs aren't appropriate for beginners. Beginners need teaching, not programs. The program begins and ends with technical proficiency.

Your athletes are ultimately the product of your skills. Would you feel proud or ashamed if another strength and conditioning coach came into your weightroom? Would you make excuses for the poor technique or accept the pats on the back for what great lifters your athletes are? The other factor—even more important than your athletes being the result of your hard work—is that your athletes are the mirror in which you see yourself. Your lifters are a direct reflection of you. When you watch your athletes, are you happy with yourself as a teacher and coach?

Technique, Technique, Technique

Never compromise. Your athletes perform parallel squats or are working to get to parallel. Don't add load until your athletes have achieved the requisite mobility to get to parallel. Gray Cook would call adding load in this situation "adding strength to dysfunction."

Our beginner athletes don't do anything but bodyweight, press-out or goblet squats to a top-of-the-thigh parallel position. In fact, we'll use 12″ plyo boxes to guarantee depth. Athletes squat to a box that places the femur parallel to the floor. Although we may need different size boxes for different athletes (or need to place pads on the boxes), we'll arrive at a point for each athlete that defines parallel for the person.

Keep in mind, these aren't Westside barbell-style box squats. The athlete touches the box to ensure depth, but doesn't relax on the box.

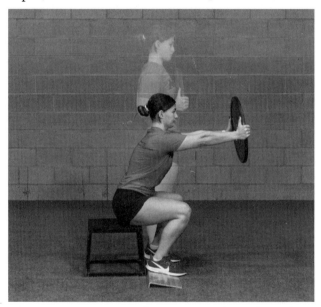

Figure 2.1—Press-out box squat, not the traditional "sit on the box" squat, but a counterbalanced tap.

Never compromise on the bench press; allow no bounce and no arch. As soon as you allow one athlete to cheat or not to adhere to the program, others will immediately follow. Remember why athletes cheat. They cheat to lift more weight, which feeds their egos. It's very difficult to stop cheating once you allow it to happen.

The late Charles Poliquin coined a term I love called "technical failure." Technical failure means you never count a rep that was completed after technique broke down. This rule will encourage your athletes to lift properly.

I regularly tell my athletes I don't care how many reps they do. I care how many *good* reps they do.

Begin with bodyweight or lightly loaded lower-body exercises, but teach basic upper-body strength exercises like the bench press.

In the first edition of this book, I strongly advocated the old idea of "bodyweight before external resistance." However, after years of training middle school kids as well as adults, I've found that concept is an oversimplification.

First, teach bodyweight or lightly loaded lower-body exercises. Athletes shouldn't squat under load if they can't squat body weight. The only exception would be the previously mentioned press-out squats or goblet squats to create posterior weight shift. Athletes must be able to get through the range of motion. It's normal to be able to squat to a parallel position. Athletes who can't squat may need additional work on hip mobility, ankle mobility or lateral hamstring stretching.

Most middle school kids won't be able to handle bodyweight upper-body exercises. I used to advocate using lots of push-ups, feet-elevated push-ups, single-leg squats and chin-ups for beginners. However, I now take a more success-based approach. Every kid learns to do barbell bench presses, assisted chin-ups (using bands) and modified suspension rows using rings because they're cheaper than buying multiple suspension training devices.

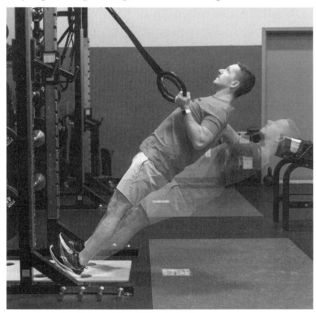

Figure 2.2—Modified ring row, a key "upper pull."

Avoid most strength tests.

The first edition of this book was written from the perspective of a collegiate strength and conditioning coach. Many of my views evolved as I began to coach primarily in the private sector.

Now here's an unpopular viewpoint: Testing is when things really deteriorate. I prefer to monitor progress versus testing athletes.

If you do testing, it should take the form of rep max (RM) tests or a heavy set done to technical failure. I no longer see the value in the 1RM tests that were such a part of my collegiate career.

Reward improvement. If you decide to test, don't simply reward strength, reward improvement. Rewarding strength is a massive mistake that encourages cheating and possibly even drug use. Rewarding progress makes athletes compete with themselves, not others.

Don't use t-shirts or record boards for rewards unless they reward improvement over personal bests. If you feel you must test strength, as perhaps in a college setting, also test performance indicators like the vertical jump and Flying 10-yard dash.

A program is only marginally effective if athletes are improving strength without changing performance factors. For certain sports, the development of size and strength is critical, but the development of size without minimally maintaining speed and power can be questionable.

Have the appropriate equipment.

This was covered in the previous chapter, but bears repeating. Many companies now sell 15-, 25-, and 35-pound Olympic bars. We've had great luck with 35-pound bars, and we now have six of these. If you're going to work with women or middle school kids, get one 15-pound bar, one 25-pound bar and a few 35-pound bars.

We also have 5- and 10-pound plastic plates the diameter of a 45- pound plate. With plastic 5s and a 15-pound bar, a middle school athlete can hang clean 25 pounds looking like a lifter. Don't underestimate the value of appearance to kids.

Success sells a program. These tools are critical for a good program. Spend money to encourage success and raise self-esteem.

Strength and conditioning coaching may seem easy in principle, but it is difficult in practice. The key to a successful program is to try to see every set and coach every athlete every day. This is time-consuming and repetitive. In fact, it's nearly impossible. At the end of a good day in the weightroom, you should be hoarse and tired.

CHAPTER 3
DESIGNING THE PERFECT PROGRAM

Program design and exercise selection are simple concepts that are usually made much more complex than necessary. You don't need to be trendy or cute in your exercise selection. In fact, after nearly 40 years of training and coaching, the basics haven't changed much. What's changed is that we now have a better understanding of why certain exercises stand the test of time.

Concepts like closed kinetic-chain exercise and functional training only serve to validate what some of the early geniuses of strength and conditioning like Bill Starr, Fred Hatfield and Ken Leistner already knew.

People who assume things about the way we coach and train at Mike Boyle Strength and Conditioning are one of the most amusing things I encounter as I travel. Because of the success of my books and the *Functional Strength Coach* video series, many people expect to find our athletes doing all sorts of outlandish exercises. The coaches who take the time to visit are surprised to see our athletes performing goblet squats, deadlifts, hang cleans and bench presses. Our athletes don't stray as far from the basics as people assume and when we do, it's for a specific reason. We'll always make changes we think will be both safe and effective.

Our job as strength and conditioning coaches is to reduce the incidence of injury *and* to enhance performance. Without an element of change, we accept the status quo. Remember the old cliché:

> *"If you do what you always did, you will get what you always got."*

Use lifts that teach your athletes to do what you want them to do. Personal trainers and coaches need to look at what they feel are the common errors of their clients and athletes and design a program that includes exercises to correct those errors. You also want to look at exercises from both effectiveness and safety perspectives, and create a program that's both safe and effective.

Good exercise selection is purposeful and designed to eliminate mistakes and correct errors.

I still like Coach Mike Burgener's (Rancho Buena Vista High School in California) "Yes to the 4th Power" idea:

> *Is it done standing?*
>
> *Is it multi-joint?*
>
> *Is it done with free weights?*
>
> *Is it characteristic of explosive sports or real life?*

We don't always adhere to Coach Burgener's philosophy, but it's a great thought process to start our programming.

Program Design Basics

The key to program design isn't to adopt someone else's philosophy, but to develop your own. Coaches shouldn't copy someone else's system. They need to do what's best, not what's trendy. For coaches to do this, they need to do three important things:

Think: What will work best for my athletes?

Question: Don't copy. Ask yourself, "Why is this exercise in my program?"

Analyze: Look for programs that get the type of result you want.

A while back, I read Simon Sinek's *Start with Why*. As we consider the preceding questions, they're about developing the WHY. Why are you doing the exercises you're doing? Great programming literally starts with *why*.

Creating a Great Program

It's imperative to have underlying goals or objectives to create a great program. Your goals or objectives should be simple and reflect your fundamental beliefs.

Strength and Conditioning Coaching

Objective One: Prevent Injuries During the Training Process

I always believed that assumption was so basic and such common sense, it didn't need to be mentioned. However, the proliferation of CrossFit® and related programs that flirt with or cross the line between safe and unsafe tells me that objective needs to be clearly stated.

To prevent injuries during the actual training process, coaches need to minimize risk. This doesn't mean *eliminate* risk, only minimize it. Everything you want to include in the program must be analyzed in terms of its risk-to-benefit ratio. Is the benefit of the exercise worth the risk inherent in it? This ratio of risk-to-benefit changes with age and level of experience. While excellent choices in general, exercises like squats, deadlifts and Olympics lifts aren't for everyone.

Training an Athlete for 18 Years

I get criticized on the internet so often, I sometimes wonder why I bother to explain myself. However, I also remind myself that I get more positive attention than I do criticism. Strangely, much of the criticism of my techniques revolves around my desire to keep our athletes healthy and injury-free. I repeatedly ask myself why so many coaches fail to see things the way I see them.

There are a couple things that are different about me and what I do. First, I'm in my 60s and have 40 years of coaching at the college and professional levels. I've also had the unique experience of coaching the same athletes for up to 18 years straight. I've seen athletes transition from healthy young men to grizzled veteran professional athletes. I've realized during this process they can still play the game, but they don't tolerate *the training* as well.

My 18-year-old collegiate athletes arrived at Boston University with young, resilient bodies. They were the filet mignon of the athletic world, the best of the best in their sport. In the 1980s and '90s—and even into the 2000s—we used squatting movements, Olympic lifts and all types of presses and pulling exercises. I'd have described us as having a relatively conventional strength program. Few athletes complained about any of these exercises being uncomfortable. Most players stayed with the same program over the course of four collegiate years. They gained size, strength and speed.

A first professional NHL season is a bit of shock for young players. The season moves from approximately 35 collegiate games to 80 games, plus playoffs. The in-season period is now almost eight months with three or four games each week. Playing 80 games plus playoffs takes a toll on the body and results in a mad dash during the summer to get healthy and regain strength.

Sadly, 100% of the players' strength is rarely regained. If I'm lucky enough to keep them for four years, most of my NHL players will find the strongest time of their careers will be the summer prior to their senior year of college. Each following summer will see them lose a little strength as the length of season, number of games and wear and tear take their toll. Around the third year in the NHL, athletes often realize their backs no longer seem to tolerate Olympic lifts and squats. Usually, this is first manifested by a small back spasm that subsides in a few days, but I learned to read the signs.

Our older, established athletes are often on a program that features trap bar jumps, kettlebell swings and lots of single-leg work. It's not that I no longer want them to do the exercises I once favored; it's the realization that these exercises are no longer suited to the high-mileage body of a professional athlete. My standard joke is that they start out like filet mignon, but finish up as beef jerky.

My job became rehab and reconditioning as my clients progressed in age. The goal is to get healthy and back in shape for the next training camp that arrives all too quickly. Most of the things I considered fundamental in their teens and early 20s are no longer relevant in our program.

Those coaches who get to train their athletes post-college experience the same things I do, but they don't often write about it.

When you choose to criticize another coach, ask yourself how long you've trained someone other than yourself. Experience counts, but experience training yourself doesn't count as much. There are too many coaches who only lift, and they fail to see firsthand the effect that playing year after year takes on a player.

Trust me, my middle school kids still do hang cleans, bench press, squats and deadlifts, but each year brings with it a "mileage" cost. The body is much like a car; the miles add up.

Becoming a Better Coach

The following are my two simple rules to becoming a better coach:

Injuries in training are our fault.

No one should be injured in training.

While speaking at a seminar more than 30 years ago, Vern Gambetta stated that coaches need to accept responsibility for injuries experienced while on a program they designed.

Hearing that was a turning point for me as a coach. Until that day, I'd have classified myself as just another meathead strength coach. I believed "real" lifters should have sore shoulders and backs. Aches and pains were viewed as a byproduct of hard training. After that seminar, I took my first step toward becoming a better coach. I made a conscious decision to make my athletes better on the field *and* to keep them healthy in training. I'm ashamed this was such an epiphany.

No one should ever be injured in training. Does this mean we train with machines and don't take any risks? No. It means we constantly balance risk-to-benefit ratios.

What we do with a young healthy 20-year-old is different than what we do with our 35-year-old NHL clients. What we do with our 35-year-old NHL athletes is different than what we do with our 55-year-old personal training clients. One size does not fit all and neither does one exercise.

This is the reason we rarely perform front squats and never do back squats or Westside-style box squats. It's also the same reason we Olympic lift from a hang position above the knees rather than from the floor. As coaches, we must constantly make choices that balance the risk-to-benefit ratio.

Objective Two: Reduce the Incidence of Performance-Related Injury

The second objective of a high-quality strength program is to reduce performance-related injuries. I used to view this as goal number one; however, recent developments in the field forced me to adjust.

Notice I used the word "reduce" and not the word "prevent." No coach or program can prevent injury. Injuries will happen—we know this. However, it's critical that we place the goal of preventing injury ahead of the goal of improving performance.

In the NFL, MLB and NHL, strength and conditioning program success is measured by the strength and conditioning coaches' ability to keep the best players playing consistently. The NHL uses a stat called "Man Games Lost;" the NFL uses "Starters Games Missed" and MLB uses "Disabled List Games." Whatever the phrase, the greatest teams keep their best players playing.

Question-Should We Fix Everything?

A guy decides to ride his motorcycle on a cold day, but right before he hops on the bike, he realizes the zipper on his leather jacket is broken. Still eager to ride, he puts the jacket on backward to break the wind. A bit down the road he hits a patch of sand, wipes out, and is knocked unconscious.

A good Samaritan arrives on the scene and starts to help.

Shortly thereafter, an ambulance arrives. The paramedic runs up and says, "What happened?" The good Samaritan says, "I found him unconscious, but by the time I was able to get his head back on straight, he was dead."

Objective Three: Improve Performance

The biggest takeaway is that your main objective isn't improving performance. We need to keep training as safe as possible. We must work to prevent or reduce in-contest injury potential. We get improved performance with that.

There are many who disagree. I can't tell you how many times I've heard coaches talk about the need to "take risks" or "lay it on the line." Those who advocate risk usually work in the area of fitness where they can brainwash clients and dispose easily of the injured. In the world of elite sport, coaches and management take training-related injury very seriously. Strength and conditioning coaches who encourage their athletes to lay it on the line in training end up in the unemployment line.

There needs to be balance. A vanilla, machine-based program without risk won't reduce the incidence of performance-related injury. The key for us is developing the ability to balance the risk-to-benefit ratio.

It's amazing how often coaches and trainers violate what I consider to be the most basic rules of program design. The information that follows isn't just my opinion; it represents a consensus among most successful strength coaches. Certain rules

Explosive Movements First

If you're using Olympic lifts or their derivatives, do them first in the program. Do exercises with high technical and neural demand at the beginning of a strength training session. I initially judge programs on this one point.

If an athlete asks me to review a program and I see the program calls for an Olympic lift after a multi-joint strength exercise like a squat or deadlift, I automatically disregard the rest of the program and usually the coach who wrote it. I feel very strongly about the basics.

Exercises that stress the nervous system as the Olympic lifts do must be done when both the muscular and nervous systems are fresh. This not only ensures the effectiveness of the lifts, but also makes them much safer. The Olympic lifts require a high degree of skill and coordination. Athletes must be fresh when performing these exercises.

Some high-level strength and conditioning coaches (most notably, Joe Kenn) have advocated intentionally performing explosive exercises after strength exercise to develop power in fatigued states. I understand the thought process, but I don't agree with it. It violates my belief in balancing risks and benefits.

Note: Now that we've moved through the CrossFit decade, performing explosive exercises for more than six repetitions is another major program flaw. At MBSC, we never go higher than five, but five versus six is splitting hairs. High-repetition Olympic lifting is a CrossFit phenomenon that needs to go away. Olympic lifts are highly technical and were never intended for high repetitions or to be used as conditioning exercises. If you disagree, ask the opinion of any knowledgeable Olympic lifting coach.

Multi-Joint Exercises Second

This concept has been stated over and over, but here's one more time for emphasis. Most coaches get this part right. Very rarely will you see a program that prioritizes single-joint exercise over multi-joint exercise in modern coaching.

Single-Joint Exercise Last…or Not at All

Most single-joint exercises are a waste of time! There are some exceptions, specifically hip and scapulothoracic work. However, exercises like leg extensions, leg curls and triceps pressdowns have little value for athletes. The time spent (wasted) on these exercises can be utilized to add exercises that have similar goals but far greater benefits.

Single-joint exercises for hinge joints like the knee and elbow simply waste time. Don't let anyone sell you on the "injury prevention" angle for things like a leg extension or leg curl. A good single-leg progression and some intelligent posterior-chain work will prevent or reduce injury incidence far better than single-joint machines.

Limit Machine Use

This is another statement I didn't think I'd have to make, but sometimes we overestimate how far the field has come. The only machines necessary in an athletic strength and conditioning program are adjustable cable columns or functional trainers. Adjustable cable columns allow rotary training (chopping and lifting actions), as well as standing row movements. Every other exercise can be done better with a weight than with a machine.

Machines that mimic conventional free weight exercises are the silliest new trend. There's a reason most machine companies have begun to manufacture benches and squat racks in addition to machines. *Space* is the best thing for a great strength and conditioning program, and machines rob a facility of space. Whenever I look at a machine, I ask myself how much use I could get out of the square footage and how many people could use that empty space.

Never Do More Than 10 Reps Unless You Specifically Want Endurance

Eight reps might even be better than 10. Spending too much time on "hypertrophy" exercises is one mistake I've made. Athletes need to lift heavy weights—and advanced athletes need to have great variety in programming. However, if the objective is strength, they need to consistently lift more. The Michael Yessis "one set of 20" concept is an exception to this rule. I've used 1 x 20 with athletes as a change of pace and they enjoyed it. For details, google "Matt Thome."

Our earlier thoughts on hypertrophy were based on flawed assumptions rising out of bodybuilding in the steroid era. Hypertrophy is generally thought to be achieved by doing a higher volume of exercise. That's a drastic oversimplification. There's a large body of anecdotal evidence that shows hypertrophy may have a genetic component. If you speak to coaches who deal with ectomorphic athletes in sports like basketball, you won't see support for the volume = hypertrophy theory. If you want to delve into this topic, look at writings on what have been classified as "hardgainers" by people like Stuart McRobert and Jason Ferrugia.

Know How Long the Workout Takes

Be realistic. I can't tell you the number of programs I've read that don't add up. Look at the time each set will take and look at the rest time allotted. I've seen programs that if done as indicated would take three hours.

Twenty sets is a good guide for an hour-long strength and power program. When you design a program, take the time to do the math, and try out the program to ensure your estimates are accurate. Allot one minute for each set and at least one minute between sets, although even that's fast. At this pace, you could get 20 sets in 40 minutes.

Tempo May Be Overrated, but Think About Contraction Type

Tempo was a big deal in the late 1980s and early '90s. If you were a follower of the late Charles Poliquin, his workouts were all about tempo. Although Poliquin gets the credit for introducing tempo to North America, Australian Ian King might have been the real innovator.

I have to admit I fell under the tempo spell for a few years. I spent a lot of time trying to get athletes to slow their eccentric contractions. However, all that tempo emphasis didn't seem to change the results, and eventually I abandoned the idea. Athletes probably just need to control the descent of the bar.

There are a couple of important points that could get glossed over when I say we no longer emphasize tempo. For long-term progress, I mix conventional concentric-focused training with eccentric and isometric emphasis. This mix might be best for advanced trainees.

However, most athletes with lower training ages don't need a mix of contraction types.

Cal Dietz has popularized what he branded "TriPhasic Training," and this may benefit more advanced athletes. However, the tri-phasic idea isn't new. Coaches like Jay Schroeder began to re-popularize isometric exercise with iso holds in the late 1990s, and the excellent work of Canadian strength coach Christian Thibaudeau made eccentric training much easier to understand and implement. Eccentric training relies heavily on the tempo concept.

Tempo is a measure of the time a repetition takes. It's usually described with three numbers, the first indicating the eccentric portion of the lift, the second indicating the time to pause at the midpoint (zero indicates a touch-and-go rep) and the last number is the concentric phase. A normal rep would exhibit a 1–0–1 tempo.

I have a few opinions on tempo:

> Normal tempo is 1–0–1. I've timed lots of lifters and was surprised that even a normal controlled rep was clearly 1–0–1.
>
> I don't love pauses because most athletes have difficulty holding a tight position during the pause, and the pause can cause unnecessary joint stress.
>
> I don't like slow concentric movements. Poliquin sometimes advocated a slow concentric contraction. I don't think this has value and we never do it.
>
> This means tempo variation is lengthening the eccentric contraction or doing some sort of isometric hold.

As I mentioned, Christian Thibaudeau came up with some excellent guidelines for eccentric training in *Black Book of Training Secrets*.

I had little success when I first tried eccentric training. The primary reason we weren't successful was that I believed what I read in the research. Research tells us that a lifter should be able to handle more weight eccentrically than concentrically. Some early estimates ran up to 120% of the concentric max. If you believe this, you're doomed to failure in your use of eccentrics.

For example, if you can bench press 300 pounds, try lowering 360 pounds (120%) under control. You'll fail miserably, and might get injured.

Most athletes couldn't do a controlled eccentric with even 100 percent of their max. What you'd see is what would best be described as an attempt at a yielding isometric, where the athlete just attempts to control the descent.

Strength and Conditioning Coaching

Athletes may eventually be able to lower more weight than they can raise, but the athletes I coached weren't even close. I don't know where the studies were done that imply athletes can lower more weight than they can raise, but it isn't true in my experience. Most athletes aren't used to lowering the bar with control; they actually lift via elasticity. As a result, they aren't able to lower the bar with control.

To develop eccentric strength, which may enhance concentric strength, Thibaudeau recommends the following:

75% 8-second lowering, 2 reps per set

80% 6-second lowering, 1 rep per set

85% 4-second lowering, 1 rep per set[1]

One way to look at eccentric training is that the number of seconds of controlled eccentric contraction should be roughly equal to the number of concentric reps you can do. If you bench press 225 for five reps, you should be able to do a controlled five-second eccentric lowering with 225.

Time Under Tension

Time under tension is the total amount of time a set takes from start to finish. Specifically, 10 reps at a 1-0-1 tempo would yield 20 seconds of time under tension. Time under tension was another well-known Poliquin/King concept. I don't worry much about time under tension, tempo or hypertrophy anymore. I do worry about technique and controlling the bar, particularly in the eccentric portion of the lift, but hypertrophy in a non-drug-using athlete will be achieved through a good program and diet. I no longer believe that bodybuilding work has much value, particularly for ectomorphic or endomorphic athletes.

We've been misled by the high responding mesomorphs of the world who'd probably respond positively to just about any type of program.

The Essential Components of a Sound Program

A sound strength program must contain all of the following qualities. Omission of any component sets an athlete up for imbalances and may eventually lead to injury or increased risk of injury.

In the simplest sense, it comes down, as Yvonne Ward says, to pushing something, pulling something and doing something for your legs.

Core Stability Exercises

Ideas on core training change often, but basically, the core is the transfer station to get force from the ground to the upper body. A vast majority of what the core does is isometric or eccentric in nature.

Core training should be focused around the prevention of unwanted motion more than the creation of motion.

In addition, sports skills are by nature primarily unilateral. The function of the core muscles (and in fact, most muscles) is different in a unilateral stance. Anyone telling you simply lifting heavy weights will promote core strength is incorrect. Lifting heavy weights in a bilateral stance won't provide anatomically correct core training.

Loaded Power Exercises

Loaded power refers to exercises like Olympic lifts, trap bar jumps, jump squats and kettlebell swings. Pieces like the Vertimax, the Total Gym Jump Trainer and the MVP Shuttle are useful tools for power development.

Medicine balls can also be used to develop total body power; however, ceiling height can be an issue.

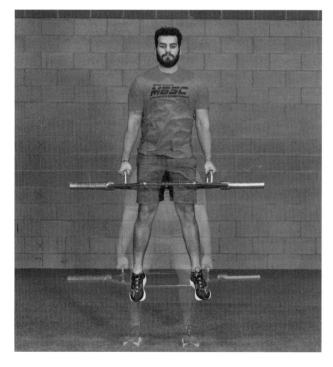

Figure 3.1—Trap bar jump, a great and simple power development choice.

---

1 Christian Thibaudeau, Black Book of Training Secrets, 2004, p40

Chapter 3—Designing the Perfect Program

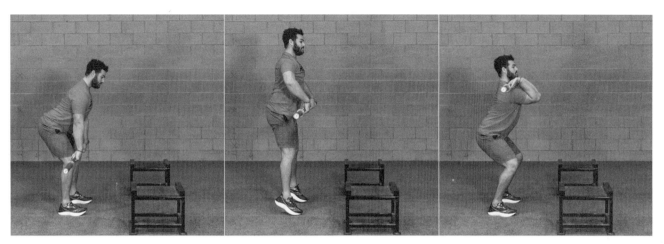

Figure 3.2—Hang clean, still a favorite, but maybe not for everyone.

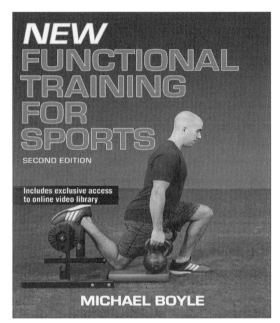

Figure 3.3—The dumbbell rear-foot-elevated split-squat as pictured on the cover of New Functional Training for Sports.

Hip-Dominant Exercises

At MBSC, the trap bar or hex bar deadlift has become our primary bilateral lift. Over the past few years, we've also begun to include more double- and single-leg hip-dominant variations. Hip-dominant exercises include bridge-based movements like slide board leg curls and different hip lift variations. We also include more glute-ham/Nordic variations, beginning with isometric holds.

I dislike the term "Nordics" and the idea of a "Nordic" leg curl. These are simply rebranded isometric or eccentric versions of a glute-ham raise, an exercise that has been around for a long time.

Also, we DON'T do bilateral hip thrusts. I'm not a fan of the bilateral version, but I do like unilateral versions. I dislike the loading position of a heavy bar across the abdomen and think most people extend the lumbar spine more than the hips.

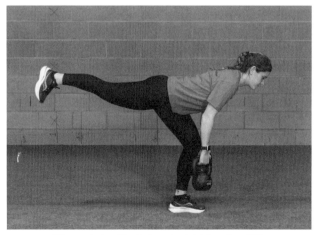

Figure 3.4—Single-leg straight-leg deadlift, a program staple for decades.

Knee-Dominant Exercises

In 2008, we made a switch to using split-squat variations as the primary knee-dominant lifts for our higher-level athletes. Now we're using more of what I classify as "single-leg unsupported" exercises, like single-leg squats and skater squats.

Beginners still do bilateral squatting primarily in the form of goblet squats, but our heavy loaded knee-dominant work will come in the form of single-leg squats, split squats and rear-foot-elevated split squats.

Strength and Conditioning Coaching

Horizontal Pressing Movements

The bench press and its many variations are frequently maligned. I like the bench press, as do most athletes. There's nothing inherently wrong or particularly non-functional about the bench press. It must be used in moderation and shouldn't be the centerpiece and focal point of a program, but this doesn't mean it shouldn't be done!

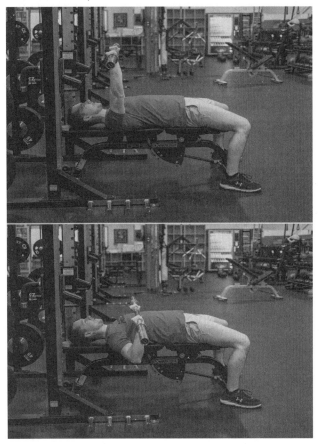

Figure 3.5—Bench press, still the best upper-body choice for those with healthy shoulders.

Vertical Pressing Movements

Vertical (overhead) pressing can be controversial. Some coaches fear overhead pressing, particularly with overhead athletes—a stance that appears somewhat paradoxical. For vertical pressing, we exclusively use unilateral versions of overhead exercises. It'd be extremely rare for us to overhead press with a fixed bar. The exception might be a younger athlete learning to lift. From a neural and coordination standpoint, younger athletes may do better with fixed bars.

In addition, we see exercises like the dumbbell incline press and landmine press as exercises that exist in the space between a horizontal and vertical press. If we think of a vertical or overhead press as pressing at zero degrees and bench press-type exercises as 90 degrees, inclines and landmines occupy the 30- to 45-degree space. Think of the landmine press as a "functional incline."

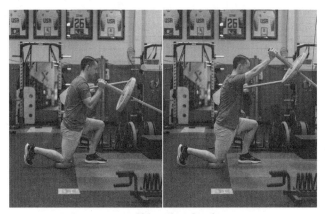

Figure 3.6—Half-kneeling landmine press, a great alternative to a conventional incline press.

Horizontal Pulling Movements

Horizontal pulling is often neglected in strength and conditioning programs. Although there are numerous options from a basic exercise like a dumbbell row to single-arm or single-leg functional versions, these exercises are often either omitted or under-emphasized.

Ring suspension rows have become our top choice in this category because they represent a scalable yet reasonably difficult horizontal entry into the bodyweight pulling category.

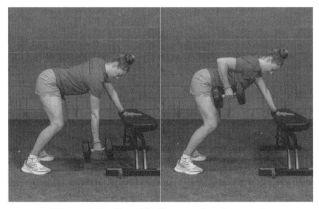

Figure 3.7—Dumbbell row, a hard to teach, hard to learn staple.

Vertical Pulling Movements

Chin-ups, pull-ups and pulldown variations make up the vertical pulling category. I'm a huge fan of chin-ups and parallel grip chin-ups for athletes. However, I find them to be too difficult for the general population.

Our athletes do chin-ups at least once per week, progressing to weighted versions, and it isn't unusual to see our female athletes performing weighted chin-ups. Ignoring vertical pulling is one of the great failings of strength and conditioning coaches today.

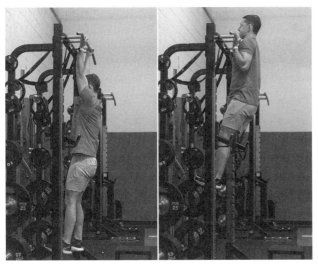

Figure 3.8—Chin-up (supinated grip), your best upper pull choice for healthy athletes.

To evaluate whether your current program is hitting all of these critical areas:

Take your phase-one program and write next to each exercise what category it would fall into.

Verify that you've covered all of the listed categories at least once during the week and preferably twice.

Look at the ratio of horizontal presses to vertical or horizontal pulls and the ratio of knee-dominant exercises to hip-dominant exercises. If these aren't in at least a one-to-one ratio, you have an unbalanced program that can potentially set your athletes up for injury.

An imbalance of horizontal presses to horizontal and vertical pulls will almost always lead to rotator cuff problems. An imbalance of knee-dominant exercises to hip-dominant exercises will lead to hamstring problems. Calculate these relationships and compare the results with your injury stats.

At the conclusion of every season, I do exactly what I'm asking you to do. I review the number and type of injuries and ask myself if everything possible was done to reduce the incidence of injury. That's how I came to many of the previous conclusions.

I still remember a year in the early 1990s when we had 20 football players with some level of rotator cuff tendonitis. When I looked at our program, I saw a typical college strength program, lots of pushing and very little pulling.

Most of our football linemen could easily bench press their bodyweight for multiple reps, but very few could do even one chin-up. I came to the obvious conclusion that our strength imbalances were at the heart of our injury issues. After forcing our athletes to perform chin-ups and assisted chin-ups, their upper-back strength increased and the rotator cuff problems disappeared.

Program design can be simple if you follow the rules. Coaches get into trouble when they program to their own likes or biases. Remember, the purpose of a strength and conditioning program is to reduce injuries *and* improve performance. As coaches, we're not trying to create powerlifters, Olympic lifters, bodybuilders or strongmen competitors. We're trying to build athletes. Strength training is simply a means to an end.

I love the Denis Logan quote, *"We want great athletes who are good weightlifters."*

I can't tell you the number of times I've had to repeat that quote over the last few years. We're trying to create better athletes; the weightroom is one tool to help accomplish that goal. For too many strength coaches, the weightroom becomes the end and not the means.

CHAPTER 4
CORE TRAINING, MOBILITY, ACTIVATION AND WARM-UPS

Core training could be a book by itself, as could mobility and warm-ups. This will be my fifth book and my fifth core training chapter, each different from the previous. In recent years, I've increasingly realized it's hard to characterize a core exercise, a mobility exercise or even an activation exercise.

Core training research and the subsequent ideas and exercises derived from them are constantly being updated. What seemed like a great idea a few years ago might be questionable now, or in some cases might be completely out of the question. I'm now totally against some of the exercises in my 2004 book. I feel like a politician, flip-flopping from side to side. For example, we no longer do any type of crunch, yet both of my first two books featured pages of crunch variations.

To make things even more confusing, core exercises have begun to creep into our strength programs. It's hard to tell when an exercise ceases to be a core exercise and shifts into a strength exercise. At what point does a lift pattern progress into what Mark Verstegen calls a diagonal push press? At what point does bridging cease to be a warm-up or activation exercise and transition into a posterior-chain exercise like a slide board leg curl? The process of core training is filled with controversy, confusion and multi-sided arguments.

This chapter will clear up some of that up for you. I'll explore the links between core training, joint mobility and the idea of "activating" muscles. These three linked ideas form a large part of what we now see as both good core training and part of a good warm-up. In fact, the best warm-up exercises are often a combination of core training, mobility and muscle activation.

Glute Activation? Is That a Thing?

To begin to understand core training and to structure a warm-up, we need to look at the key compensation patterns that occur when we move.

Dr. Stuart McGill uses the term "gluteal amnesia" to describe the inability to properly use the glutes. In a warm-up, we might use an activation exercise to attempt to "awaken" the gluteal muscles. However, as with so many things in this field, the idea of muscle activation drills has come under fire. The reaction to the volume of activation drills has been a typical overreaction, sending us in the opposite direction.

Because coaches have over-simplified and said things like, "Your glutes are shut down," it provides room for controversy and disagreement. Let's make this clear: As long as muscles have nerve flow, they're "on."

But just because a muscle works doesn't mean it works optimally. For example, substituting lumbar extension for hip extension is the major culprit in many of the athletic back problems we see today. People often do what's easy, not what's ideal.

As we look at athletes, both injured and healthy, the inability to properly use the glutes relates to at least four major injury syndromes:

Low-back pain strongly relates to poor hip extensor activation—poor glute function will cause excessive lumbar compensation.

Hamstring strains strongly relate to poor glute max activation—think about the concept of synergistic dominance.

Anterior hip pain strongly relates to poor glute max activation—this relates to the poor biomechanics of hamstrings as hip extensors.

Anterior knee pain relates strongly to poor glute medius strength or activation.

Shirley Sahrmann believes that anterior hip pain can be the result of poor glute function and the resulting synergistic dominance of the hamstrings.[2]

---

2 *Shirley Sahrmann, Diagnosis and Treatment of Movement Impairment Syndromes, 2001, p15*

Sahrmann discusses the simple biomechanical explanation by citing the lower insertion point of the hamstrings on the femur. If the hamstrings are consistently called upon to be the primary hip extensor, the result will be anterior hip pain in addition to hamstring strains. The anterior hip pain is a result of the poor angle of the pull of the hamstrings when used as a hip extensor.

Sahrmann makes one of her many lucid points:

> "…when assessing the factors that contribute to an overuse syndrome, one of the rules is to determine whether one or more of the synergists of the strained muscle are also weak. When the synergist is weak, the muscle strain is probably the result of excessive demands."[3]

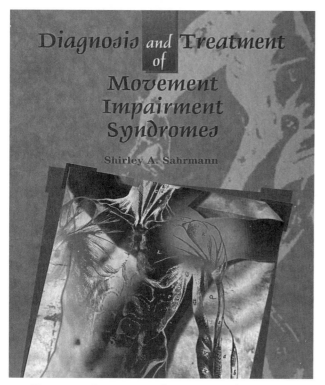

Figure 4.1—Diagnosis and Treatment of Movement Impairment Syndromes—*you can read the first sections over and over.*

I call this "looking on the roof." If you see water streaming into your house, you don't simply plug the hole or paint over the water stain—you look for the source of the water; you look on the roof for the problem. The same applies to injuries. Don't focus on the pain site; focus on the pain *source*. In our athletes, the source keeps coming back to the glutes (or maybe the lack of glutes).

In the bigger picture, coaches should look at every non-traumatic, non-contact injury as having a root cause in either poor program design, weakness of synergists…or both.

We generally perform some type of basic glute activation drills at the beginning of every workout to develop better awareness of the function of the glutes and to hopefully "wake them up" so they'll be greater contributors to the workout.

One small problem: When does hip extension work become resistance training versus core training? There's a thin line between hip-dominant exercise and core training. The solution may be to do some core work as a warm-up (quadruped and bridging), and progress these concepts into hip-dominant strength exercises.

In describing the core, Dr. McGill uses the analogy of the core as "a fishing rod held up by guide wires." In other words, the spine is a flexible structure made stiffer or more stable by outside influences. McGill has also described the deep abdominal muscles as drawing strength from crisscrossed layers, much like plywood. Both analogies may help outline our picture of core training.

McGill's work is both interesting and compelling, and his books, *Back Mechanic* and *Low Back Disorders,* are must-reads for any strength and conditioning professional.

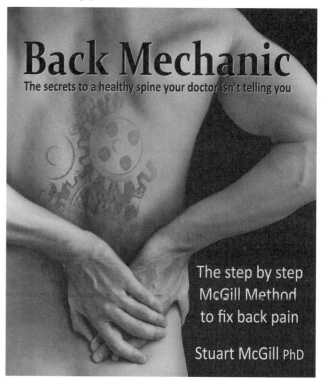

Figure 4.2—Back Mechanic, *a "must read."*

---

3   Shirley Sahrmann, Diagnosis and Treatment of Movement Impairment Syndromes, 2001, p37

Another complementary analogy to the fishing rod is to see the core muscles functioning like the lines or rigging of a sailboat. Think of the spine as a mast, pretty much useless without sails and rigging. Add the rigging and sails (abdominals, obliques and nearby musculature) and the sail can be controlled for movement and rigged for speed. The lines control the movement of the sail to harness the power of the wind. The sail is useless without the mast and the mast is useless without the sail.

Similarly, the core muscles transfer the power of the lower body to the upper body through its system of rigging. Think of this rigging as anti-rotators and stabilizers for both the sail and mast. The lines don't just move the sail; they also harness the power of the wind.

Our ever-expanding knowledge of functional anatomy has shown that the abs don't really pull the ribcage toward the pelvis as in a crunch. The function of all of the abdominal muscles might be better seen as *preventing* or controlling motion rather than *causing* it.

Back to the rigging of the sail idea: The anterior core muscles connect and position the pelvis and ribcage to harness and transfer power from the legs. Without muscular control, the spine develops "energy leaks." Well, wind with no sails or rigging is just wind.

Our increased understanding of functional anatomy has brought words like "anti-extension," "anti-rotation" and "anti-lateral flexion" into our training lexicon. This increased understanding was in large part due to the work of people like Shirley Sahrmann, James Porterfield and Carl DeRosa, as well as Dr. McGill.

Sahrmann states:

"During most daily activities, the primary role of the abdominal muscles is to provide isometric support and limit the degree of rotation of the trunk…A large percentage of low back problems occur because the abdominal muscles are not maintaining tight control over the rotation between the pelvis and the spine at the L5–S1 level."[4]

In other words, the abdominals generally do a poor job of controlling rotation—of anti-rotation. They are poor rigging.

Sadly, many advocates of powerlifting or Olympic lifting feel that most of the scientific advances made in the areas of sports medicine and physical therapy don't apply to strength sports. As with many points made by those who consistently lift weights with two feet on the ground, on this we disagree.

I believe our influences in the area of core training should be the researchers, doctors and physical therapists who deal with injured athletes, not the people from the sports of powerlifting or Olympic lifting who are sending their injured lifters to these influential doctors and therapists.

It seems easy for those Olympic lifting and powerlifting coaches who never have to worry about athletes running or jumping to tell us how to train those who do. Unfortunately, when these coaches begin to move from strength and power development into the performance enhancement world, problems arise. But science can't be denied… at least not for long.

Science tells us that the deep abdominal muscles (internal oblique, external oblique, transverse abdominus and multifidus) play a key role in the stability of the lumbar spine. Many in the strength community seem to disagree. Although disagreement is healthy, I've seen far too many strength athletes with problems in the hips and low back for me to believe that exercises like squats and deadlifts provide enough core stability training. If this was true, no conventional lifter would ever experience back pain.

> *Athletes and clients must learn to move from the hips, not from the lumbar spine.*
>
> *I believe that most athletes with lower back pain or hamstring strains have poor hip and/or lumbo-pelvic mechanics and as a result, they must extend or flex the lumbar spine to make up for movement unavailable through the hip.*

Learning to stabilize the spine and move the hips—hip *mobility* in the presence of lumbar *stability*—is probably the key to being able to strength train while remaining healthy. Thirty years ago, I didn't understand or appreciate the functional anatomy of the deep abdominal musculature or the functional anatomy of the hip. Although I'm now well-versed, I continue to study and learn about these critical areas.

Most recently, people like Ron Hruska and the Postural Restoration Institute® (PRI) have added

---

4 *Shirley Sahrmann, Diagnosis and Treatment of Movement Impairment Syndromes, 2001, p71*

another layer to our ever-evolving understanding of the core.

For years, we contemplated how to stabilize the spine. Dr. McGill and Paul Hodges proposed different stability strategies. In the first edition of this book, I wrote extensively about the Australian methods of training the deep abdominal muscles.

The work of Richardson, Hodges and Jull, through their landmark work *Therapeutic Exercise for Spinal Segmental Stabilization in Low Back Pain,* significantly advanced our knowledge of core anatomy and core muscle function. That book, and the research preceding it, changed the way core training was both perceived and performed. Years later, after McGill's *Low Back Disorders,* coaches and therapists debated bracing versus drawing in as we sought to understand how to access and utilize what were effectively "new muscles" to many of us.

> ### Terminology
>
> **Drawing in**—the action of bringing the rectus abdominus toward the spinal column. Theoretically, this is done by contracting the transverse abdominus, external oblique and internal oblique muscles.
>
> **Hollowing**—another description of a drawing-in action that assumes the action results in a decrease of waist diameter. In hollowing, the goal is to get as thin as possible.
>
> **Bracing**—the technique taught and favored by McGill that involves a simultaneous co-activation of the transverse abdominus, internal oblique, external oblique and rectus abdominus. In bracing, there's no attempt to decrease the diameter at the waist, only to co-activate the muscles.

In strength and conditioning at the time, these disagreements primarily came down to semantics. The Australian/Hodges research in the area of drawing in may still be applicable to athletes, but whether it's a draw-in or a brace may be slightly less relevant than initially thought.

Although I'm clearly not qualified to dispute Dr. McGill's research, I do have a small point of theoretical disagreement. McGill's research shows that drawing in or hollowing can decrease the base of support and stability of the spine. However, if we're teaching a drawing-in action as a neuromuscular awareness exercise but not as the primary vehicle for stability, does that present a problem? McGill himself states, "Hollowing may act as a motor re-education exercise."

The PRI folks use what we called a "quadruped draw-in." They now call it an "all-four belly lift." It's kind of a *Back to the Future* thing.

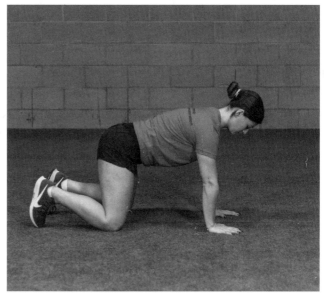

Figure 4.3—Quadruped position, a great place to start a core program.

Breathing and Core Training

Breathing is where we really missed the boat in core training. I failed to understand that intentional breathing—what we might call "deep breathing" or "diaphragmatic breathing"—has a significant muscular component.

In fact, although breathing is reflexive, not all athletes breathe properly or fully utilize the correct muscles. Our core training program now begins with breathing, and intentional breathing is incorporated into nearly every core exercise.

We now know, primarily from studying PRI, that the critical deep abdominal muscles needed as stabilizers are also breathing muscles. As we study breathing, we see the transverse abdominus, internal oblique and external oblique classified in the breathing world as muscles of "end-stage exhalation." In other words, aggressive exhalation is facilitated by the deep abdominal muscles. The deep abdominal muscles assist as air is forced out.

Google "the value of blowing up a balloon." You don't need to blow up balloons; you only need to understand the end-stage exhalation involvement of the deep abdominal muscles.[5]

In core training, we can use this to our benefit, using forced exhalation as a method to help recruit the deep abdominals. Instead of telling athletes to draw in or brace—what we'd now consider an "artificial" cue—we cue them to execute a maximum exhalation. This exhalation will naturally recruit the stabilizers we attempt to "turn on" in core training. The difference in how to do core exercises now comes down to breathing. The concept of the exercise remains the same, but the isometric contraction of the deep abdominals we sought to elicit with verbal cues is now fueled by a hard exhalation.

This leads us to the author David Epstein's idea of "neglected connections" and "undiscovered public knowledge." In his book *Range* (p180), Epstein describes how there's often readily available information from a seemingly unrelated discipline.

Nowhere is this more evident than in the study of breathing. For decades, the review of breathing was left to respiratory therapists and yoga teachers and was completely neglected and in many cases even rejected by the strength and power community. In the past, when asked about breathing and breath work, I'd often jokingly reply, "All my clients are currently breathing." At the time, I thought I was clever, but I now realize I was very dumb.

This relationship of breathing and the core musculature explains the concept of the ki-yi in judo, which is to use a shout to help break a fall, and probably also explains the many grunts we hear on the tennis court. Major point: A hard exhale aids in the stabilization of the core and the recruitment of the deep abdominal muscles.

Suddenly, breathing became a critical piece of the core stability puzzle. In the past, most coaches didn't care how their athletes breathed, only caring that they were breathing. We may have argued about breathing in versus breathing out or about breath holding, but never about the action itself.

The first key to understanding breathing is to recognize that the diaphragm is a muscle and although it will work involuntarily, it can also be consciously engaged.

In "good" breathing, the diaphragm works during inhalation and the deep abdominal muscles work during exhalation. On inhalation, there's a concentric contraction of the diaphragm.

In effect, the diaphragm is a dome that flattens on concentric contraction and pushes down on the abdominal contents. This is why deep breathing is often referred to as "belly breathing." To create a visual picture, I like to use the analogy of kids at camp playing with a parachute, pulling the parachute down.

We also now understand that a breath should come in through the nose to facilitate the diaphragm to descend. An athletic exhale should be hard and through pursed lips, like blowing out candles.

The diaphragm is a muscle! That light bulb went on when Sue Falsone was doing an in-service lecture at Mike Boyle Strength and Conditioning and said the diaphragm was her favorite muscle. I sat there thinking, "The diaphragm is a muscle?" Then I remember wondering, "How do we train a muscle we can't see or touch?"

Here we sit thinking about inhaling—yes, the diaphragm is the yin to the deep abdominal yang—to facilitate one muscle and then exhaling to facilitate others. Suddenly, the idea of core stability training makes more sense. The research was pointing toward facilitating the deep abdominals to create the stability we sought. However, instead of saying "brace," "draw in," "pull your belly button in," all we need to say is "exhale hard" and "exhale long." That was a major light bulb moment.

Inhale through the nose, moving air down into the ribcage. We want no shrug on the inhale because a shrug means athletes are using accessory muscles of inspiration—think scalenes, levator, SCM.

Athletes should exhale out of the mouth as if blowing out candles. I tell my athletes to exhale like they're at my birthday party and need to blow out more than 60 candles. Blow out hard and blow out long. To facilitate this, most of our core training uses five-second concentric isometric contractions.

Then…What Is Core Training?

To go back to the first paragraph of this chapter, the areas of warm-up, muscle activation, core training and mobility become hopelessly intertwined.

Sahrmann refers to the idea of "the right muscle moving the right joint at the right time." A better description in the core stability world might be "the right muscles stabilizing the right joint (or joints) at

---

5   *https://www.ncbi.nlm.nih.gov/pmc/articles/PMC2971640/*

the right time." In either case, this is one of the most simplistically brilliant statements ever written and is central to our concept of warm-up, mobility and core training. We want the right muscles moving the right joints at the right time—the right muscles stabilizing the right joints to help make this happen.

This means parts of the warm-up may be basic mobility exercises that include a core training component. Exercises like double-leg bridges, single-leg bridges, leg lowers and floor slides have a combined focus on mobility, muscle activation and core control. The goal of getting "the right muscle moving the right joint at the right time" is the true goal of a warm-up for us.

The glutes should extend the hips while the core musculature controls or limits lumbar extension. It means the hip flexors should control leg lowering while the core muscles prevent lumbar extension.

The key to core training is the realization that we're working on multiple components. Gray Cook might refer to this as developing "motor control."

With core training, we may not even be strengthening, but instead are reeducating the neuromuscular system. To do this, the athlete needs the ability to isometrically control the core while concentrically and eccentrically using the glutes and hip flexors.

WHAT TO DO?

The Updated Essential Eight— Eight Drills Everyone Should Do

Building on the original "A Joint-by-Joint Approach to Training," my article based on a conversation with Gray Cook, this is an update on a follow-up piece I called "The Essential Eight." The initial version was a list of eight simple exercises everyone can and should do to warm up. This version will simply update that idea with a few notable changes.

The nice thing about these exercises is that anyone can do them. Everyone may not be able to do them well, but they can do them. The people who can't do them well obviously need them the most. Don't let people talk you out of warm-ups.

We can hide mobility under the heading of "warm-up" or "stretching." It's like hiding a pill in peanut butter for a dog—it makes it much easier to swallow. Some people call these mobility drills.

Others call them activation drills, and some might just call it part of the dynamic warm-up. I like to think, "D: All of the above."

Number 1—Thoracic Spine Mobility

The mobility of the thoracic spine is one of the least understood areas of the body and was previously the realm of physical therapists. Physical therapist Sue Falsone might be singlehandedly responsible for introducing the athletic world to the concept of thoracic mobility and, more importantly, for showing the world of strength and conditioning some simple ways to develop it.

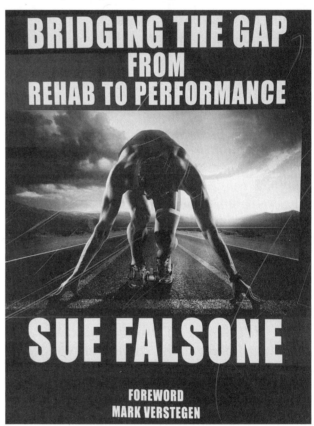

Figure 4.4—Bridging the Gap from Rehab to Performance.

One nice thing about t-spine mobility is that while almost no one has enough, it's pretty hard to get too much. We encourage our athletes to do thoracic mobility work every day. To perform our favorite thoracic mobility drill, all you need is one of the new Rollga foam rollers.

It's increasingly clear that these Rollgas are going to make the regular foam roller obsolete. The Rollga has grooves and ridges, so the bone has a void to fit into—in the case of the t-spine, it's the spine or more specifically, the spinous process. This allows greater penetration into the soft tissue.

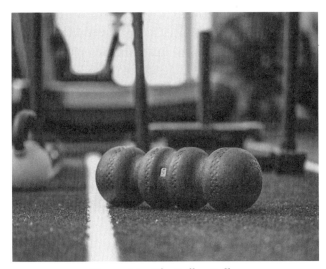

Figure 4.5—The Rollga Roller, a game-changer in the soft tissue world.

To roll the thoracic spine, begin with the roller at the thoracolumbar junction and work up to about C7. We do a bit in flexion with the hands behind the head and the chin to the chest, and some in extension with the hands overhead. The Rollga roller allows the spinous processes to fall into the groove and effectively provides an anterior-to-posterior mobilization of the vertebrae with every roll. Have your athletes take some time to breathe through each rep.

Once again, I have to admit I was wrong about the effect of the breath on mobility and core training—considerably wrong. I used to make fun of yoga practitioners and anyone else who brought up breathing. But as it turns out, there's a big difference between breathing and breathing correctly. Watch for your clients to inhale through the nose (called "nasal inhalation") and exhale through the mouth.

This drill is done as part of our foam rolling sequence. The rest of the mobility work is done after we put the rollers away.

Number 2—Neck Mobility

The idea of neck mobility sounds bad. I get it—you hear "neck mobility" and think about scenes from the old horror movie *The Exorcist*, where the possessed girl's head spins in circles.

This drill might be better referred to as "*slow and controlled cervical spine range of motion,*" but that makes for a lousy headline.

This is actually an idea stolen from Tim Anderson's Original Strength group and is simply quadruped head turns and nods. These are gentle! It isn't trying to push for a greater range of motion; it's simply getting the neck moving.

BIG TIP here from Anna Hartmann: Do your neck ROM while trying to look at your nose. Yes, look at your nose. Looking at your nose creates the necessary chin tuck.

The drill is five turns right and left for 10 total, and 10 nods up and down, all with the eyes looking at the nose.

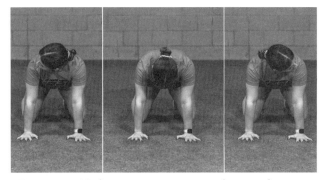

Figure 4.6—Neck rotation, active cervical range of motion.

Number 3—V-Stance T-Spine

The Rollga roller provides the anterior-to-posterior t-spine mobility work, while the V-stance t-spine drill works rotation. Admittedly, I discovered this technique entirely by accident. In this drill, we're combining a stretch (the V-stance split-stretch) with a t-spine rotary mobility exercise. It's just a reach, exhaling throughout the reach.

The V-stance really locks down the pelvis and forces the rotation to come from higher up the spine.

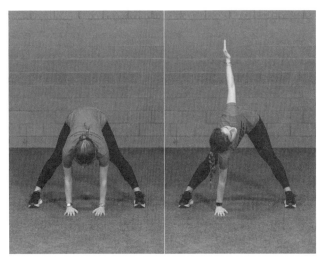

Figure 4.7—V-stance t-spine, anchor the hips, reach and look.

Number 4—Double-Leg Bridge

This is a supine exercise. Did you have to stop for a second to picture that? I like to remember how to visualize "supine" using a somewhat grim analogy. They used to bury people in pine boxes on their backs. Gross maybe, but it always helps me remember "supine."

The supine progression teaches people to use the glutes while maintaining core position using the deep abdominal muscles.

Bridging is an exercise that checks the three boxes of mobility, activation and core training. A bridge is a hip mobility exercise (hip extension), an activation exercise for the glutes and, when properly done, also activates the anterior core muscle. These "three check" exercises now form the basis for our warm-up and are part of our core training.

To perform a double-leg bridge, you'll have your clients begin in a hook-lying position with the feet flat on the floor and knees bent. Then they'll dorsiflex the ankles to get the toes off the ground and drive through the heels.

This dorsiflexion action can be a bit controversial. Some coaches prefer to drive through the whole foot. However, driving through the heels better facilitates the hip extensors. Our experience has shown that "quad dominant" athletes (I hate that term, but it probably applies here) will actually push into the floor with the balls of the feet in a leg-extension type movement to lift the hips off the floor. They'll complain they don't feel their glutes but do feel low-back pressure.

"Toes up" tensions the entire posterior chain.

With the toes up (dorsiflexed ankles), they'll drive the heels into the floor to raise the hips. The goal is to create a straight line from the knee through the hip to the shoulder. The big key is to create and maintain this posture by using the glutes and hamstrings, not by extending the lumbar spine.

This is where we bring in more concepts from Postural Restoration. Think about keeping the ribs down so the rib cage and pelvis stay in alignment.

The two-bowl analogy some coaches use is a helpful visual. Imagine the pelvis and rib cage as two separate bowls. The goal is to keep the two bowls positioned over each other. My introduction to this was when watching Boston Bruins strength coach Kevin Neeld's *Optimizing Movement* video lecture.

Any drop in the hips drastically reduces the effectiveness of the exercise. The key here—and the key to all the core exercises I use—is to exhale as hard as possible while contracting the glutes and raising the hips. The hard exhale creates abdominal tension and most importantly, it does it naturally.

In our current core program, we use five-second isometric contractions combined with five-second hard exhales. One rep is one five-second hold. During that hold, we have the athletes focus on a hard exhale. The key is to have them think about squeezing the glutes as they blow out through pursed lips.

Remember, hard exhales from the mouth recruit the deep abdominal muscles. When we do any core exercise, we cue a forceful five-second exhale on the concentric contraction. Instead of counting reps, we count exhales. It ends up being the same, but the emphasis is entirely different. Instead of saying, "Do a set of five-second isometric holds," we cue, "I want five reps of five-second exhales." As they bridge, we tell our athletes to blow out like they're blowing out birthday candles.

One exhale is one rep. Program these in five five-second exhales.

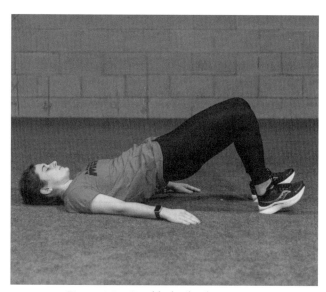

Figure 4.8—Double-leg bridge, toes up, heels into the floor.

Number 5—Single-Leg Bridge

We follow double-leg bridges with single-leg bridges. The key here is to simultaneously drive the heel into the ground and the knee toward the chest. Look for co-contraction of the hip flexors on one side and the hip extensors on the other.

The same "five-second exhale" idea applies.

For time efficiency, do three "reps" of five-second exhales on each leg. Cue to drive the heel into the ground, think about contracting the glute and exhale hard while counting to five. This is a valuable exercise that again provides a triple emphasis on the glutes, hip flexors and on the deep abdominals.

The single-leg bridge amps up the glutes and hamstrings and also teaches the critical difference between hip and lumbar spine ranges of motion.

This ability to distinguish between hip and lumbar spine motion is one of the most important goals of our supine exercises. In many exercises that target the hamstrings and glutes, it's easy to mistakenly use more range of motion at the lumbar spine than at the hip.

In addition, it's easy to extend the hips with the hamstrings instead of using the glutes.

The single-leg bridge can be seen as both an exercise and a test. If an athlete performs the exercise and experiences cramping in the hamstrings, it's an indicator of weak glutes or inhibited glute function.

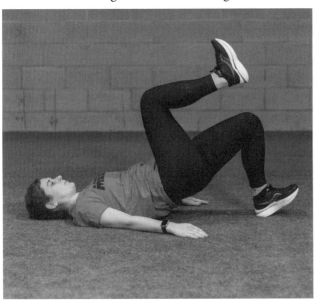

Figure 4.9—Single-leg bridge, flex the opposite side hip past 90 to limit lumbar compensation.

Have your client start by holding a knee to the chest and then progress to an active hip flexor contraction with a tennis ball held in the flexed hip "pocket." The tennis ball must not fall. When extending from the lumbar spine instead of the hips, the ball will fall out. This means the athlete is inadvertently substituting lumbar spine motion for hip motion.

Gray Cook popularized this exercise to teach athletes how to separate the function of the hip extensors from the lumbar extensors. Most athletes are unaware of how little range of motion they possess in the hip joint when the lumbar spine motion is intentionally limited. As you watch this, you'll quickly realize the range of motion in this exercise might only be two to three inches.

The range of motion can be significantly increased by relaxing the grip on the opposite knee, but that defeats the purpose. Relaxing the hold on the leg simply substitutes lumbar spine extension for hip extension.

> **Why Do the Hamstrings Cramp?**
>
> In hip extension with the knee bent, the hamstring muscles should be a weak synergist. Due to its shortened nature, the hamstrings should provide a small measure of assistance to the glutes in hip extension. However, in the absence of good glute function (McGill's gluteal amnesia), the hamstrings are forced to become the prime mover. Attempting to be the prime mover while shortened causes the muscle to overwork and cramp.

Number 6—Leg Lowers

Leg lowers are another great exercise that hits mobility, core work and muscle activation. I describe leg lowers as "the most complicated single-joint exercise you can do." To a novice, a leg lower looks like a lying hamstring stretch. However, to do a leg lower properly requires core control and control of both hips.

The movement starts supine with both legs raised and as the name describes, one leg is lowered toward the floor. Doing this correctly requires eccentrically using the hip flexors of the lowering leg, the deep abdominal muscles as stabilizers (hard exhale) and the extensors of the down leg to keep that leg flat.

We program three five-second lowers on each leg, cueing "blow your leg down" to emphasize the hard exhales.

Strength and Conditioning Coaching

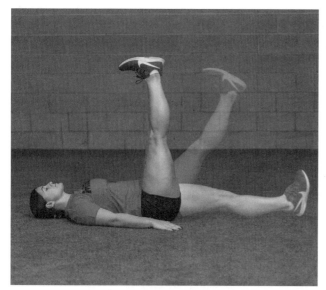

Figure 4.10—Leg lowers, start with both legs up; lower one down, keep the up leg straight.

Number 7—Floor Slides With Breathing

I have to tell you, I love floor slides. Talk about bang for the buck. Floor slides:

- *Activate low trap, rhomboid and external rotators*
- *Stretch the pecs and internal rotators*
- *Decrease the contributions of the upper traps*

Try these slides with your athletes and be amazed. Here's one thing that might convince you: Some of your clients won't even be able to get into the position. This isn't unusual. Asymmetry in the shoulders will be another surprise. A third surprise might occur when your athletes try to slide overhead—many will immediately shrug. This is dominance of the upper trap. Keys to the floor slide:

- *Scapulae are retracted and depressed*
- *Hands and wrists stay flat against the floor—hopefully the back of both hands can touch the floor*
- *Have your athletes think about pressing into the floor with the forearms*
- *Don't let them go past the point of discomfort. You'll notice the anterior shoulder will release and the range of motion will increase—don't force things.*

The big key is a hard exhalation on the way up. Cue to think about blowing their hands up.

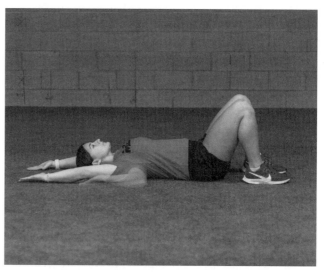

Figure 4.11—Floor slide, press into the floor while exhaling.

Number 8—Mini Band Walks

The original idea from the "Essential Eight" article was to add an upper-body component to mini band walks and to have the band in the hands. The only problem was that many people didn't retract the scapula; instead, they shrugged...and activated the wrong stuff.

So, we simply went back to the old mini band idea. It's okay to use regular mini bands, but we've gone with a more heavy-duty version made by Slastics and sold as Safety Toner Loops by Perform Better. These last for years.

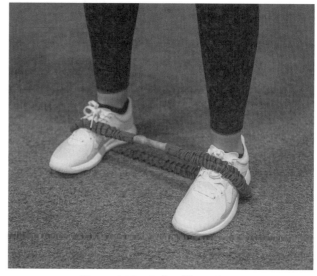

Figure 4.12—Safety Toner Loop, a super durable mini band from Perform Better.

We do a series of double-leg abduction and external rotation, single-leg abduction and external rotation, and the old stand-by, lateral walks.

Core Exercises?

In some ways, almost every exercise can be seen to have a core component.

Years ago, flexion exercises were designed with core strength in mind. The thought was that a strong front equals a healthy back. However, looking at training through our functional anatomy lens, we see the need not for flexion of the spine, but for stability and rotational control.

The "crunching" act of bringing the shoulders toward the hips never happens in athletics or even in normal life. My standard joke is someone might perform two crunches a day: one to get out of bed and one after a nap, and even that's a stretch.

Modern core training breaks into anti-extension, anti-lateral flexion and anti-rotation. The initial emphasis is simply on the prevention of movement with simple isometric exercises. These exercises are then progressed by either adding motion or by changing the base of support.

Strangely, in the topsy-turvy world of core training, suddenly even planks are under fire as not being functional. What? We still plank and side plank with beginners and younger athletes. It's difficult to see how good, old-fashioned core stability can be a bad thing.

Anti-Rotation Training

Anti-rotation training is the most recent controversial area of core training. Anti-rotation has come under fire from internet "experts" who don't seem to understand the principle. The contrarian argument is that rotation is natural and shouldn't be prevented or restricted. They fail to see that the goal of anti-rotation exercises is not to stop rotation, but to *control* rotation.

Anti-rotation exercises develop the capability to control the rotary forces so critical to sports, and aid in the transfer of forces from the ground to the hands. Think of this as "thickening the ropes that control the sail." Flimsy ropes tear, control is lost and in the worst case, the mast (the spine) is damaged.

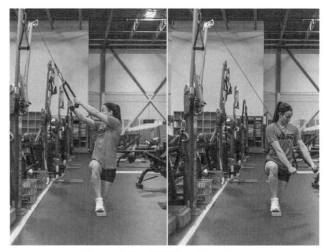

Figure 4.13—Half-kneeling chop, high to low in the frontal plane.

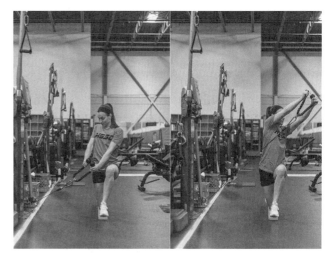

Figure 4.14—Half-kneeling lift, low to high in the frontal plane.

The concept of chopping and lifting patterns as exercises was first introduced to the athletic world by Gray Cook. He advocated diagonal patterns of trunk flexion with rotation (chop) and trunk extension with rotation (lift).

His 1997 article, "Functional Training for the Torso," was a quantum leap in our training thought process. He was one of the first to advocate combining the concepts of conventional strength training with the approaches in rehabilitation to effectively produce a new category of strength exercise: rotary exercise.

Cook described sequences of chopping and lifting moving from a kneeling or half-kneeling position into a standing position. Kneeling or half-kneeling is initially used to allow focus to be on core control. The idea was, in his words, "to eliminate joints." Positions like tall-kneeling and half-kneeling limit hip, knee and ankle movement and let the lifter focus on the core control aspect of the exercise.

He has since modified his original versions, shifting the chop and lift exercises into exercises in which the arms transfer force in a diagonal pattern through a more stable torso. In his eyes, the concept of rotary training involves stabilizing the trunk while moving through a diagonal, rotational pattern.

Chopping and lifting patterns involve movements primarily in the frontal plane that force the person to isometrically control rotation as the load is moved through the frontal plane. The exercises can both challenge and develop trunk stability through the use of a cable column or functional trainer.

Athletes must be able to prevent rotation before we allow them to produce it.

The action of moving through a chopping or lifting pattern prior to a rotary component is a necessary precursor to the actual patterns of chopping and lifting. Athletes must be able to isometrically resist the forces of rotation before those forces can be used in a propulsive manner.

Performance enhancement expert Mark Verstegen probably deserves the credit for moving Gray Cook's concepts onto the field through his work at Athletes' Performance™, the predecessor to today's EXOS™ facilities.

In the Athletes' Performance philosophy, rotary training was viewed as a program component much like squatting or pressing. It's now common, but it was an industry-changing idea at the time.

Anti-rotation training is a blending of core training and strength training, as well as a blend of conventional strength training thoughts with insights from physical therapy. In our MBSC rotational training, we primarily use Keiser Cable Columns, Functional Trainers and Ancore Trainers to create diagonal loads or to load diagonal patterns.

We can trace the roots of rotary and anti-rotation training further back to Dorothy Knott and Margaret Voss and the diagonal patterns of proprioceptive neuromuscular facilitation (PNF).[6] Although we now recognize PNF more as a neuromuscular stretching technique, the original idea was far more extensive.

Knott and Voss advocated diagonal patterns of exercise involving both sagittal-plane prime movers and the muscles responsible for transverse and frontal-plane control.

Physical therapists noticed these diagonal patterns of extension and rotation are a vital part of movement and started to use them to provide a more "real world" aspect to rehab. Specialists in rehabilitation realized that movement was multi-planar and that the highest form of rehabilitation would involve diagonal patterns of flexion and extension combined with rotation.

Thomas Myers, in his book *Anatomy Trains*, describes what he calls the spiral and functional lines of the body, while Vladimir Janda made us aware of the integrated workings of the musculature across the critical junction from the glutes to the opposite-side lat. This area, known as the thoracolumbar fascia, along with the hip joints, allow us to move force from the ground out to the extremities.

These diagonal patterns were initially termed "chopping and lifting" patterns. Many early attempts at rotary training butchered these patterns. Chopping is best viewed as a pattern of flexion and rotation, but in the beginning stages, it's probably not best illustrated by the actions of chopping wood. Instead, think about moving a load through the frontal plane (high to low) in the presence of a stable core. In order to better facilitate this, our half-kneeling position has progressed to an in-line half-kneel.

We eventually realized the position of the front foot and back knee mattered more than we initially thought. As athletes progressed in load, stances became wider and the exercises moved more from stability to strength exercises as the base of support was widened to allow greater loads.

We added an "in-line" component to return these exercises to lighter loads with more of a stability emphasis. We utilize small, orange "balance beams" we get from Perform Better, but 2 x 4s will certainly do just fine. The goal is to have the foot and knee in line to force a narrow base of support.

The lift is a pattern of extension and rotation with a focus on, as Sahrmann says, "movement occurring at the shoulders." Chop is the reverse and is a flexion and rotation pattern.

Neither pattern actually involves significant trunk flexion or extension but rather are stability exercises. Initially, both exercises were taught from

---

6 https://www.amazon.com/Voss-Knotts-Proprioceptive-Neuromuscular-Facilitation/dp/0397548605

Chapter 4—Core Training, Mobility, Activation and Warm-Ups

the half-kneeling position. In the lift, the inside knee was down, while in the chop, the outside knee was down.

However, as we began to look at throwing sports, we altered our leg position to more closely resemble a throwing action, dubbing this version the "in-line pitcher's chop." This resulted in confusion as to what was right or wrong. We now realize that both options in chopping (inside knee down, inside knee up) can be correct. It really depends on the specific adaptation you're looking for.

Half-Kneeling Lift

- *Have your client assume a split-squat position on the balance beam. The inside knee is down. (Note: We've recently begun to explore what you might call "semi in-line." This means the knee is on the beam and the foot is outside but touching the beam. Some of our coaches feel the balance component is too restrictive and I think I agree.)*

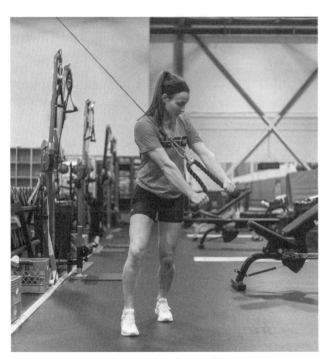

Figure 4.15—Semi in-line foot and knee position.

- *A triceps rope is held to the side and the eyes are focused on the hands.*

- *The action is a two-part "pull to the chest, push over the opposite shoulder." We're explicit about the "pull it in, push it away" aspect.*

Half-Kneeling Chop

- *Have your athlete assume a split-squat position on the balance beam. The inside knee is now up.*

- *A triceps rope is held to the side; the eyes are again focused on the hands.*

- *The action is the same concept of a two-part pull and push, but now the instruction is "pull to the chest, push down and away." We're still explicit about "pull it in, push it away."*

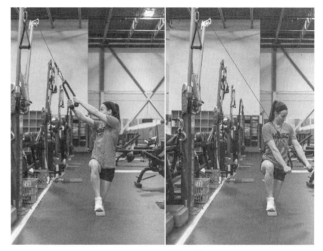

Figure 4.16—Half-kneeling chop.

In-Line Pitcher's Chop

- *Your client will assume a split-squat position on a balance beam. The inside knee is now down.*

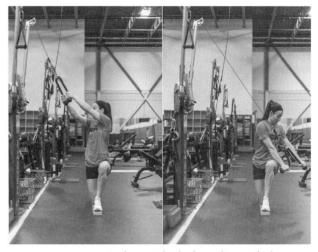

Figure 4.17—In-line pitcher's chop, this might be a more "functional" version.

55

Strength and Conditioning Coaching

- *A triceps rope is held to the side and the eyes are again focused on the hands.*

- *The action is the same concept of a two-part pull/push, but now the instruction is "pull to the chest, push down and away." We're still explicit about "pull it in, push it away."*

- *This change in leg position now more closely replicates the rotary actions of throwing.*

It's worth noting that Cook initially intended for these exercises to be done with a bar about four feet in length. This required the inside leg to be down in chopping so the bar could clear the leg. Staying inside knee down was the classic "that's the way we've always done it" thing we often criticize.

Dynamic Chop and Lift

The dynamic chop-and-lift patterns now move to a standing position and become multi-joint extension and rotation or flexion and rotation exercises. The emphasis is on teaching an athlete to transfer force from the ground through the trunk and into the hands in the diagonal chop-and-lift patterns. Mark Verstegen described the standing lift pattern as a "rotational push press."

To perform the dynamic standing lift:

- *Your athlete will grasp the triceps ropes with the thumbs up.*

- *Position your client perpendicular to the cable column with the feet slightly wider than shoulder width.*

- *The lifter begins in a squat position with the hands outside the leg closest to the cable.*

- *The action is now "stand, rotate, press" in a rapid, fluid motion. The hands move from the machine side of the body to an arms-extended position on the opposite side. The key is to take the patterns learned in the half-kneeling or lunge position and make them explosive.*

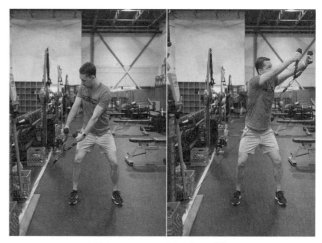

Figure 4.18—Standing lift, Verstegen's "rotational push press."

To perform the standing chop:

- *You'll begin with the triceps rope attachment set as high as possible.*

- *Have your client grasp the rope handles with the arms extended and the eyes looking at the hands.*

- *Cue to think of the "pull-push" action of the half-kneeling version, but this time it's done rapidly. Don't think about "chop" as much the idea of pushing an opponent to the ground.*

Transverse Chop

We also began to experiment with a pure sagittal version we dubbed "transverse chop." A transverse chop is again a "pull-push" action but is done strictly in the sagittal plane. This is probably one of the most "sport specific" or "sport imitative" exercises we do in the weightroom. When done well, transverse chops look like a baseball swing or a hockey shot.

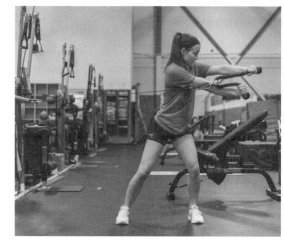

Figure 4.19—Transverse chop, sagittal plane power.

Anti-Lateral Flexion

Our anti-lateral flexion progression generally goes side plank, side plank row and suitcase carry. We've now added a side plank with adduction, more commonly known as "Copenhagen planks" or "Copenhagens."

Here we are, adding one more entry into the geographical lexicon. First, it was Romanian deadlifts, then Bulgarian lunges and Nordic leg curls. But now we have cities claiming exercises, with Copenhagen getting its own adductor exercise. Much like its geographical predecessors, the Copenhagen adductor exercise or Copenhagen plank is now the current cure-all for groin strains. What is it with geography and injury-prevention claims?

In case you're not familiar with it, the Copenhagen adductor exercise is a modification of a side plank designed to create both concentric and eccentric stress on the adductor muscles.

To be honest, it's better than I originally thought. My initial impression upon seeing online videos was to worry about the valgus stress on the knee. However, after numerous trials and no complaints of MCL pain or discomfort, that concern was put to rest.

Another issue is that much like a multi-hip machine, this is a long-lever, frontal-plane adduction. In the world of functional anatomy, adduction and abduction are concepts, not actions—they never really happen!

Pure frontal-plane adduction never occurs, particularly with a straight lever arm. All true adduction involves either a hip-flexion component (like the recovery stride in skating or striking a soccer ball) or a hip-extension component (as in a crossover).

Let's also be wary of any exercise that's presented as a panacea. One thing we can be certain of is that training helps prevent injury. Study after study has shown this. As a result, using Nordic hamstring exercises will decrease hamstring muscle injuries and adductor strengthening exercises will decrease groin injuries. And just about every lower-body intervention ever studied decreased the incidence of ACL injuries.

The lesson here isn't specific—it's general: Training will aid in injury prevention. Better exercise choices will produce better results, but progressions and regressions are key. The Copenhagen plank is a

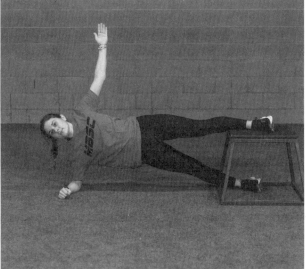

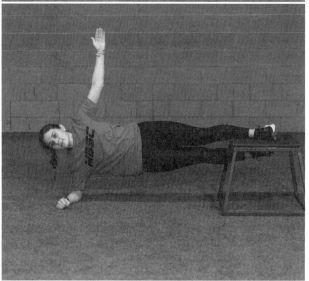

Figures 4.20—Copenhagen plank, incorporating adductors and lateral stabilizers.

nice progression of the side plank, so it can certainly be part of an integrated core arsenal. The flip side is that we want to utilize the Pilates ring, cables and sleds that still comprise our adduction program.

Straight-Leg Abduction

If you have access to a Pilates Reformer or the new Glute Slide, a standing straight-leg abduction is another excellent exercise to strengthen the glute medius. Simply have your athlete stand on the Reformer or Glute Slide with one foot on the base and the other on the pad, and attempt to abduct. This exercise is especially difficult because momentum can be minimized and the spring or elastic resistance is increased in the end range.

Conclusion

Hopefully, this chapter has made you rethink core training. To me, core training is at the center of the "functional versus non-functional" and "isolation versus integration" arguments.

I've been on both sides of this argument, and my work over the past few years has totally changed my position. As stated previously, I believe many athletes can't properly use the glutes or abdominals. These inabilities are at the heart of many dysfunctions ranging from low-back pain to hamstring injuries.

Some degree of isolative core work seems essential to "rewire" these neural patterns and correct dysfunctions. It's clearly not beneficial to return to just single-joint exercises, but isolative work in the core is a necessity.

From core stability to core strength, to hip stability and into rotary training, our approach to training is rapidly changing. The days of uniplanar, rectus-dominant abdominal work are clearly gone and are being replaced by an ever-evolving series of exercises emanating primarily from the world of physical therapy. Keep an eye on this in the future and be open to changing your thinking as new concepts appear and research develops.

CHAPTER 5
EXPLOSIVE TRAINING

"Olympic weightlifters are athletes;
athletes aren't Olympic weightlifters."
~ Michael Boyle

"We want great athletes
who are good weightlifters."
~ Denis Logan

This chapter is about explosive training under load, where we're talking about Olympic lifts and variations, kettlebell swings, jump squats and trap bar jumps. This is training for the wires—the nerves. Don't think about explosive strength. That's a bit of an oxymoron; think about explosive power. We may work a lot of muscles in explosive training, but that's not the main point.

I know I keep going back to the beer and chocolate chip ice cream idea, but just remember that explosive training isn't about what someone likes. Think about developing explosive power, but more importantly, think about picking the right tool for the job.

I often use the "chainsaw analogy." Imagine if a carpenter showed up to work on your house with nothing but an 18-inch chainsaw—probably not a good choice for installing crown molding. A lot of coaches are like the chainsaw guy. They have one tool and they want to use it for everything.

If you don't like Olympic lifting, that's okay. Everyone doesn't need to Olympic lift, but most of our young athletes do. On the flip side, most of our pros don't. Just pick a way to be explosive. But Olympic lifting is fun, safe and challenging when done correctly and aggressively supervised. Work with your athletes on developing great technique and bar speed, and put less emphasis on the amount of weight lifted.

The key to quality Olympic lifting is that it should look good. I use what I call the "crap" test—substitute any word you like. Simply put, if it looks like crap, it probably *is* crap. I can walk into any weightroom in the country and tell how good the coach is simply by watching the athletes. If they can't lift, that coach can't or won't teach. Either is a problem.

The proper use of Olympic lifts and their variations will lead to improvements in power and athleticism that you might not have thought possible. You'll be amazed at how proficient your athletes will become at lifts you may have initially felt were too difficult to teach or learn.

Before We Get Too Far...

Remember this:

If you can't teach a lift,
don't use it in your programs.

This is the type of common sense statement I wish I didn't have to make in 2025. This applies to all areas of a program, but it particularly applies to Olympic lifting. If you can't teach the Olympic lifts, don't use them. Period. You don't necessarily need to be able to perform the Olympic lifts under load, but you've got to be able to teach and demonstrate them at least with an unloaded bar.

Using lifts you're unable to successfully demonstrate and teach is a classic strength coaching mistake. The reason many sports medicine professionals and sport coaches feel the Olympic lifts are unsafe is because strength coaches frequently place these exercises into a program without proper instruction and without constant supervision.

If you can't teach and supervise your athletes in the Olympic lifts, get your high-velocity hip extension training from things like trap bar jumps, jump squats, medicine balls and plyometrics. Learn to balance the theoretical benefits of Olympic lifting with practicality and safety.

Many coaches allow athletes to Olympic lift in an unsupervised environment and as a result, athletes might get injured due to lifting with poor technique. Before adding explosive movements to your program, learn to teach the movements. Don't worry about weight; worry about technique.

An exercise like the hang clean is no more responsible for an injury than a car is for a car crash. Cars are safe when driven as directed; hang cleans, hang snatches and other Olympic variations are safe when done as directed. Problems usually lie with the instruction and supervision, not the exercise.

Olympic lifting requires constant supervision, so even if you're capable of teaching the lifts, ask yourself how much time you can spend in the weightroom actually teaching and coaching. If you're prepared and have the time to teach, by all means, add Olympic movements to the program. Your athletes will see great gains in power and will probably learn to enjoy the athleticism of Olympic lifting more than they enjoy conventional strength work.

Years ago, I asked legendary University of Minnesota skating coach Jack Blatherwick why he didn't have his athletes Olympic lift. His explanation was simple. He said, "Mike, I'm not always around when the guys lift and I don't want them doing a complicated exercise like the clean on their own." Pretty simple.

Make intelligent, informed decisions. Don't just do stuff because everyone else does.

Why We Clean

Recently, some of my former interns and assistants participated in a discussion about performing rack pulls versus hang cleans as a power development exercise. Some coaches supported the idea of using rack pulls as a substitute for hang cleans; however, at Mike Boyle Strength and Conditioning, we remain "clean" people. At MBSC, we still see numerous benefits from performing the Olympic lifts we feel may not be achieved as well with alternatives.

Why We Don't Clean From the Floor

In my mind—and in our MBSC programs— Olympic lifts are used for power, and trap bar deadlifts are for starting strength or strength off the floor. If we want to improve starting strength or strength from the floor, we'll load the bar in the trap bar deadlift.

If we want power, we'll Olympic lift from a hang-above-the-knees position or do weighted jumps. The key is to always choose the right tool for the job. We've Olympic lifted from the hang-above-the-knees position for nearly 30 years. My feeling has always been the pull from the floor is simply a deadlift that gets the bar into the proper position to perform the hang clean. When we begin to attempt to Olympic lift for starting strength, we again confuse issues or cross wires. We're choosing the wrong tool for the job.

In addition, the hang clean is a great equalizer. The standard Olympic plate is 450 mm in diameter (slightly under 18″). This means taller athletes are at a mechanical disadvantage when Olympic lifting from the floor. This makes them more prone to back injuries due to the increased amount of hip, knee and trunk flexion needed just to get into the start position. Lifting from clean blocks from the hang position allows athletes to compete on a level playing field, experience less back stress and have a lower chance of injury.

Power Production

The evidence is strong that Olympic lifting results in improvements in explosive power. We've documented athletes who increased their vertical jump by a foot in our training programs (yes, 12 inches). Can these results be attributed solely to Olympic lifting? Probably not, but we're convinced Olympic lifts play a huge part in increased power production.

High-Rep Olympic Lifting?

In spite of what the CrossFit crowd tries to tell us, high-rep Olympic lifting is generally not regarded as safe. One of my biggest disagreements with CrossFit (yes, I have a few) is the use of high-rep Olympic lifts. Olympic lifting is a power development tool, not a conditioning tool and not a muscle endurance tool. You can bang in a nail with a screwdriver…it just takes a lot longer to get the job done.

Using Straps

I love teachable moments. These are the times I realize we have a philosophy at Mike Boyle Strength and Conditioning that may not be familiar even to those who work there. In our staff meetings, I find myself saying, *"I've said this 100 times, but probably never to this group."*

I stole that line from Coach Jack Parker at Boston University. He would always say, "I've said _____ in team meetings for 30 years, but maybe not to this team." As our staff changes, I find I assume everyone knows everything about what "we" believe. Then I get snapped back to reality.

Vertical Jumping as Monitoring

Monitoring is hot. We've got HRV, Omega-wave, morning resting heart rates, questionnaires and more. Logically, we all want to know our athletes' training status. Are we doing too much? Are we doing too little? Is it planned overreaching with hopes of a supercompensation effect or are we just beating them up day in and day out?

With the rise in popularity of CrossFit, it's not uncommon for people to work to failure and then cheat to get beyond that in search of a training effect—often multiple times per week.

Years ago, when we were still doing an off-season Combine/Pro Day program, we started doing weekly vertical jump tests. Initially, this was because we were practicing vertical jump for the upcoming testing days. But I began to see it as a monitoring method.

Initially, I wasn't sure what the variability would be and how an overtraining effect would show up. I quickly realized a three-to-five percent change was significant from a training standpoint. Five percent is only one-and-a-half inches off a 30-inch vertical jump, but a drop from 30 to 28.5 probably indicated we'd overtrained or, as my man Brandon Marcello likes to say, under-recovered.

The key in looking at the three-to-five percent drop-off is to put it in terms we're more familiar with. From a pitching standpoint, three to five percent would indicate a drop from 95 mph to 90–92. This would be cause for concern.

In the 40-yard dash, the time would rise from 4.5 seconds to 4.72 with a five percent change. Again, this is a cause for concern.

A Monday decrease from the previous week is a strong indicator that we need to deload or at least decrease volume, or maybe both.

There does seem to be some post-activation potentiation (PAP) effect in certain athletes, but not all athletes. To define post-activation potentiation:

"The underlying principle surrounding PAP is that prior heavy loading induces a high degree of central nervous system stimulation, resulting in greater motor unit recruitment and force, which can last from 5 to 30 minutes."[7]

We've seen increases after our first one or two sets of a strength exercise. We may do two or three sets of vertical jumps for monitoring purposes. Set one (three attempts) is usually done at the end of a warm-up that includes medicine ball throws and plyometrics.

In one non-scientific study, we saw significant increases in vertical jumps done after a conditioning workout. In that case, we tested the vertical jumps of our Boston University hockey players and had some disappointing results. Players then did a fairly difficult treadmill sprint interval workout of 10/10 sprints. These are uphill sprints done at a 10% grade and 10 mph. Players returned from the treadmills and jumped 10% (three inches) higher in some cases.

This may prompt further study into the potentiation/activation idea.

In any case, vertical jump testing can be a great way to get a quick check on the status of the nervous system at the beginning of the week to look at training effects off-season or recovery in-season.

---

7 Chiu, Fry, Weiss, et al., 2003; Rixon, Lamont, & Bemden, 2007

Back to straps: As I watched a young female client struggle with a heavy set of hang cleans, I said, "We need to teach her to use straps; her problem is her grip, not her hips." She responded that an MBSC coach had instructed her to put the bar down between reps, to rest and regrip. I was shocked. I thought, "Who the heck would say that?" But, it was one of our own coach's words. Lack of communication is always the head coach's fault, so the blame was on me.

My thought immediately went to, "Have we ever talked about straps as a staff?"

Probably not.

Here's the policy: Straps are for advanced lifters.

You'll see when athletes begin to struggle to hold the bar and seem to be concentrating as much on grip as on the lift. This is when we introduce straps. The bottom line is to not limit lower-body power because of a lack of grip strength. That makes no sense.

We don't teach a hook grip. We don't tell them they need to concentrate. We don't tell them they need additional carries to work on grip. We teach them to use straps.

In that case, the primary goal is power development. Straps undoubtedly help that. Let's make sure we all learn how to use straps and how to teach athletes to use them. They may initially regress, but they'll thank you later. Two tips:

Straps are always "under the bar first, over second."

Force athletes to learn to adjust straps with only one hand. I can't tell you how many times I watched an athlete use the right hand to adjust the left strap and then be unable to wrap the right side.

Athletes should be able to flip the straps "under-over" and "roll them in" with the same hand! Flip the strap over and pin it with your thumb. Then roll the bar to tighten it.

Straps are a game-changer when introduced at the right time. Your athletes will look at you and say, "I can't believe we didn't do this before."

Straps can also be an exercise in frustration. Encourage athletes to use them on all warm-ups until they're proficient with them.

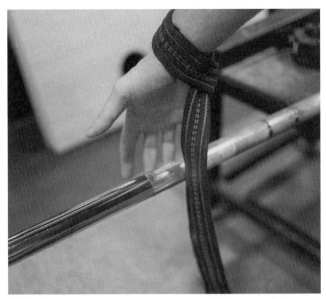

Figure 5.1—Straps under/over, the key to straps is that they go under the bar first and then over!

Teaching the Olympic Lifts

The easiest way to learn and teach the Olympic lifts is from a high hang position. In fact, every good Olympic lifting coach I've seen speak or whose work I've read advocates a "top down" approach.

You're trying to improve an athlete's performance at his or her sport, not trying to produce weightlifters for the Olympics. We keep coming back to the Denis Logan quote that we want to produce "great athletes who are good weightlifters."

The hang position with the bar above the knee eliminates a great deal of the lower-back stress often associated with the performance of Olympic lifts. Any size athlete can become a great technician from the hang position.

However, many athletes due to height or inflexibility will have difficulty learning the lifts from the floor. The physiological characteristics that make great Olympic weightlifters (good lever system, mesomorphic body type, great hip flexibility) aren't present in many of our athletes. I often tell our basketball players and rowers that the exact qualities that make them good basketball players or rowers make them poor candidates for competitive weightlifting.

Let's look at some numbers. These may be less accurate for larger athletes like football linemen and obviously don't apply to younger high school athletes. Football linemen generally don't have great strength-to-bodyweight ratios or power-to-bodyweight ratios.

Chapter 5—Explosive Training

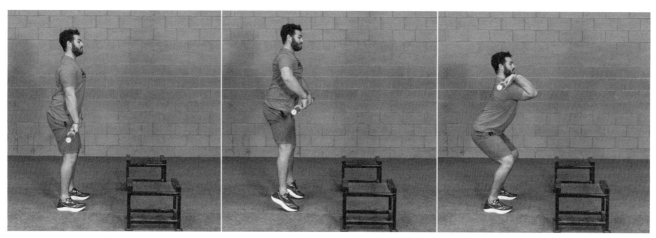

Figure 5.2—Hang clean sequence—Our big "Pendlay change" is to start from position one. We now start higher on the thigh when teaching.

Strength-to-power ratio is another area to consider. Many athletes have a large strength focus and a poor strength-to-power ratio. Strength to power is simple: Just look at a trap bar deadlift versus a hang clean.

A double-bodyweight deadlifter should be able to hang clean in the 1.3 to 1.5 range.

EXCELLENT	GOOD	FAIR	POOR
1.5 x BW	1.3-1.4 x BW	1.1-1.2 x BW	1 x BW
Ex 300 Hang Clean @200 lbs	260-280	220-240	200

*Hang Clean to Bodyweight Relationship
(Advanced Male Athlete)*

EXCELLENT	GOOD	FAIR	POOR
.9 x BW	.8 x BW	.7 x BW	.6 x BW
Ex 180 Hang Snatch @200 lbs	160	140	120

Hang Snatch to Bodyweight Relationship

A Quick Cleans Teaching Checklist

Good explanation (under 20 seconds) and good demo (two or three reps)

Flat back picking up the bar

Hands-free front squat—learn to carry a bar on the deltoids

Front squat—learn the front rack position

Position one: shoulders back, arms long, wrists curled under

Cue "jump, shrug, sit"

Elbows up in the catch

Back flat returning the bar

I find myself constantly saying, "Jump up, sit down." Try it, it works.

Many Olympic lifting purists don't like the "jump" cue. Guess what? It works great. I think those purists do more harm than good with relentless nitpicking of athletes on social media these days. Keep repeating "We want great athletes who are good weightlifters."

I also always find myself decreasing weights and telling kids, "I don't care how much weight you move, but I do care how fast you move it."

> **Pendlay Position One**
>
> A quick note about what we now call "position one." Several years ago, I encountered a gem from the late Glenn Pendlay's teaching progression that I felt could improve how we teach the hang clean or the hang snatch. Instead of attempting to teach athletes to hinge or to slide the bar down the thighs, Pendlay would instruct the lifter to slightly bend the knees.
>
> This slight knee bend creates enough hip and knee flexion to put the lifter in a good start position for what we used to call a "high hang" clean. It also eliminates the difficult concept of teaching the hinging effect needed to slide the bar down the thighs. Instead of creating a hinge—a forward lean—the athlete simply bends the knees.
>
> I know this may seem simple, but this was a game-changer for us in teaching.
>
> Quick note: Just bend the knees. Don't lean back. Weaker kids will lean back to use body weight to counterbalance the weight on the bar. The chest should be just over the bar…or ever so slightly behind.

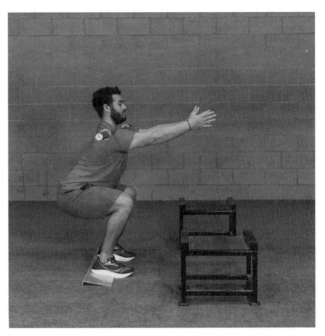

Figure 5.3—Hands-free front squat, teaching an athlete the bar needs to be supported by the anterior deltoids and collarbone.

Hang Clean Alternatives?

Many coaches don't feel comfortable teaching the Olympic lifts, but obviously still desire increases in hip and leg power. For these coaches, trap bar jumps and dumbbell jump squats may be the answer.

Although I'm a big proponent of the hang clean, we see athletes at the college and pro levels who don't have enough upper-body flexibility to properly rack the bar in the clean position. This results in sloppy attempts to perform the hang clean and clean variations.

Some strength and conditioning coaches propose using dumbbell cleans as a solution for athletes who don't possess the flexibility to properly rack (or "catch" if you prefer that term) the clean. Unfortunately, I haven't found that dumbbell cleans allow an athlete to handle appropriate amounts of weight. In addition, a dumbbell clean teaches a "reverse curl" bar path that's not desirable in quality Olympic lifting.

The kettlebell clean is another alternative. But I'm not a fan of kettlebell cleans or snatches either. I know, Joe Kettlebell will use my logic against me: It's all in the teaching, right? Sorry, you won't win me over with that argument. I will only say that I have found athletes are not patient enough to learn kettlebell cleans and kettlebell snatches.

As an initial result of my dislike for some of the proposed alternatives, I've begun to use trap bar jumps with greater frequency for athletes who aren't suited for or proficient at the Olympic lifts.

Using the Trap Bar Jump

I love trap bar jumps. I wish I could say who gave me the idea because I'd love to give credit. (I think it was Arizona Coyotes Director of Performance, Devan McConnell.)

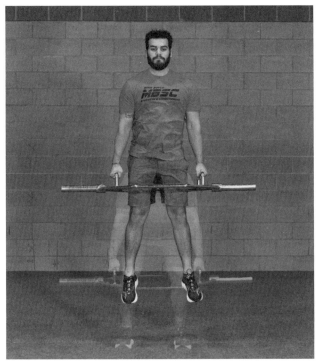

Figure 5.4—Trap bar jump, a great alternative to the hang clean.

In any case, to properly discuss trap bar jumps, we need some context. All our athlete programs other than our baseball program ideally begin with some variation of an Olympic lift. However, every year in our summer pro hockey group, we have a number of athletes who've never trained with us and are either unfamiliar with Olympic lifts or don't want to Olympic lift.

This means we need an alternative explosive exercise. In some cases, we did additional jumps, in other cases kettlebell swings—and in others, we used our MVP shuttle.

However, when we started to trap bar jump, this quickly became our go-to exercise for power with athletes who weren't Olympic lifting.

Before we get too carried away, let's talk a bit about how we do these. Our "why" is explosive power development, but "how" can get a bit fuzzy.

Our idea of how to do trap bar jumps evolved, in a round-about way, from the work of JB Morin (via my friend Cam Josse). JB's actual work was in sled sprinting, but if you bear with me, you'll see how the two ideas mesh.

JB and others like Matt Cross and Pierre Samozino have spent years investigating the correct way to determine loads for sled sprints. To make a long story short, JB's extensive research led him to conclude that the sled load should result in a time that's 150% of the unloaded time at the same distance. This means the correct load for a guy who runs a 1.5-second 10-yard dash is a load that causes him to run a 2.25-second 10-yard sled sprint.

The key point is that load isn't based on body weight—it's based on how the load effects speed. Morin refers to this as speed decrement and aims for 50%. More on this will follow in the speed chapter.

We simply adopted the same idea for the trap bar jump. To load trap bar jumps, we selected a weight that would allow 60–70% of the athletes' best vertical jump. To calculate this, we do the exercise on our Just Jump mats and compare. A load that generates a jump less than 60% of the best vertical jump is deemed too heavy. To me, this seems simple. Athletes who can vertical jump 30 inches use a load that will produce a jump of 18–21 inches.

Unfortunately, we often see loads based on a percentage of body weight or on a percentage of the best trap bar deadlift. These are both bad ideas.

Using a percentage of body weight seems like a safe and simple idea until you start to evaluate larger athletes. Larger athletes in general will have less relative strength. A load of 30% of body weight might be fine for a 200-pound player (meaning 60 pounds), but terrible for a 300-pound player at 90 pounds. In fact, in general, heavier players should get lighter loads, not heavier.

Using a percentage of the best deadlift is even worse because this assumes a direct relationship between strength and power that doesn't exist. I'm thinking of two similar athletes in our facility, both with 36″ vertical jumps. One is highly experienced in the weightroom, with a trap bar deadlift max in the 500-pound range. The other has struggled with back problems and hasn't trap bar deadlifted over 275 pounds. Does it make sense to load them differently based on strength…or similarly based on power?

Interestingly, both could vertical jump over 25″ using 95 pounds on the trap bar. The correct load in both cases wasn't based on body weight or strength, but on how the load affected power output. Take a few minutes, and give this a try. I'm positive you'll fall in love with the idea the same way I did.

Jump Squats

Jump squats have been popular with European track-and-field athletes for years. Jump squats provide a great deal of the hip power many athletes seek from Olympic lifting, and are perfect for athletes who have reservations about technique or athletes with shoulder or back problems that prevent them from Olympic lifting.

I've never been a big jump squat person (maybe out of concern for the cervical spine), but I plan to investigate jump squats more as an alternate to trap bar jumps. We have begun to use dumbbells more as this eliminates the cervical compression/impact and the potential shoulder external rotation restrictions.

To perform the jump squat, your athletes will simply jump from a position that approximates an athletic stance or a half-squat.

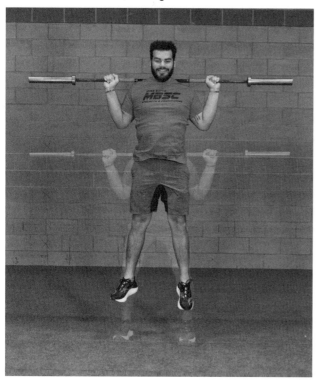

Figure 5.5—Jump squat, another Olympic lift alternative.

Beginners can land and stabilize between jumps, while more-advanced athletes can utilize a plyometric response off the floor.

The most important issue for jump squats is again load selection. Authors and researchers have recommended using a percentage of the back squat 1RM as a load, most often using 25 percent. Much like with trap bar jumps, this method of loading is flawed and potentially dangerous, as it again doesn't take into account the athlete's body weight.

To calculate load, you can simply use the aforementioned Morin/Josse method if you have a jump mat. The load is appropriate when the athlete hits 60-70% of his or her best vertical jump.

In any case, whether you choose to develop leg power through Olympic lifting, trap bar jumps or by performing jump squats, the use of external loads to train the legs and hips can be the fastest way to achieve gains in lower-body power.

The beauty of Olympic lifts and weighted jumps is that the athlete can build power without developing large amounts of muscle. The training emphasis is on the nervous system, not the muscular system, making this an excellent training method for athletes such as figure skaters, wrestlers and gymnasts.

Many athletes and coaches have the mistaken impression that explosive lifting is only for football players. This couldn't be further from the truth. Olympic lifting and its variations are suitable for athletes in all sports and of all sizes, and should be of particular interest to athletes looking for total-body strength without increases in size.

Snatches and Dumbbell Snatches

Snatches are easy to teach—easier than cleans. I think most coaches disagree with this statement, but I also believe the coaches who disagree have never tried to teach their athletes to snatch and don't use snatches in their programs. Those who disagree simply haven't tested my hypothesis.

My reasoning is simple. The greatest obstacle to overcome in learning to clean is upper-body flexibility. Many athletes, particularly those who've been on a "mirror-oriented" program, will have decreased flexibility or mobility in the shoulders, elbows and wrists. To perform the snatch, you don't need to be as flexible in the shoulders, elbows or wrists. You simply need to be able to get your arms over your head.

If I encounter an athlete who can't get into the proper catch position for the clean, I go right to teaching the snatch and forget about the clean. Often if I have athletes who've experienced low-back pain, I'll only use snatches or trap bar jumps for power work. Snatches will generally use loads of 50 to 60 percent of the athlete's hang clean, and as a result will place much less stress on the athlete. In addition, for many athletes, the finish position of the snatch places less stress on the low back than a tight athlete trying to raise the elbows into the proper position to catch the clean.

Dumbbell snatches also get a bad rep, but I don't know why. I love the dumbbell snatch as a power variation. From an athletic standpoint, the asymmetrical nature of the lift makes it an excellent choice to increase core and shoulder demand.

Kettlebell Snatches

Although I'm a dumbbell snatch fan, I'm not a kettlebell snatch fan. I've had numerous discussions with people in the kettlebell community about this, most of which became acrimonious. But I believe the time needed to perfect the kettlebell snatch and the wrist discomfort encountered during this time make it a poor choice for group training.

The kettlebell proponents love to argue that people quickly adapt, but our experience didn't bear that out.

Single-Leg Olympic Lifting

The following thought has been a long time coming. In fact, it might be close to 30 years in the making. The initial impetus for this came from Jeff Oliver, strength and conditioning coach at The College of the Holy Cross. In the early 1990s when Jeff was my graduate assistant at Boston University, we attended Vern Gambetta's Building the Complete Athlete weekend course. We both returned with a new appreciation for the concept of single-leg training, and we implemented much of what we learned. Our programs were progressive and innovative for the time, and are probably still better than what many coaches do today.

I remember Jeff jumping on the platform to do a few single-leg hang cleans. His rationale was, "If single-leg squats make so much sense, why not single-leg cleans?" My reaction was to call him crazy.

Fast forward about 20 years, and we're doing almost exclusively unilateral exercises in the weightroom. Why not single-leg Olympic lifts? Why's it taking so long to embrace single-leg Olympic lifts? I could come up with a number of rationalizations. They look weird? Athletes will react negatively to these bizarre new exercises? My resistance to single-leg Olympic lifts was just like everyone else's reaction to single-leg strength work. Truth is, I was acting just like the people I was encouraging to change.

Seeing the concept in action eventually triggered the move. In the summer of 2010, Boston Bruin Patrice Bergeron was a visitor in our BU weightroom. I was intrigued as I watched Patrice effortlessly single-leg hang clean 135 pounds for five and then proceed to do 180 for five in the same fashion. I went over and asked who taught him this, and he said his strength and conditioning coach in Quebec. Patrice's demo showed me the bilateral deficit I'd spoken so strongly about in strength was also clearly evident in power. Now, I don't know Patrice's 1RM hang clean, but I can safely assume it was less than 300. However, his 180 single-leg clean for five reps showed another illustration of bilateral deficit.

I had one small problem. I needed a group of good Olympic lifters to test my theory. Fast forward to 2013: My US Hockey Women's National Team became just that group and from day one, they didn't disappoint. I asked the players to do five reps at 50% of their normal loads, and they did so with ease. We did single-leg hang clean, single-leg hang snatch and single-leg/single-arm dumbbell snatch. In all cases, the bilateral deficit was evident. Athletes who struggled to do 135 for five could easily do single-leg cleans with 70 for five. The snatch results were even more glaring. Molly Schaus easily single-leg barbell snatched 55 pounds for five with a projected 1RM of about 110.

However, it's now 2025 and we still haven't implemented them. The latest push came from a discussion with Dan Pfaff, where in an X/Twitter discussion, Dan said:

"They are a staple for me at all levels and all sports. I typically use them at the end of the week to reduce injury risks that exist with normal Olympic lifts. They are also a constant plan B with leg injuries."

You know I love this quote:

"If you have not changed your mind about something in the past year, check your pulse, you may be dead."
~ Frank Gellet Burgess

Mark Verstegen loves to use the term "logic train." So…take this logic train with me. We've embraced single-leg strength in our programs. For years, we've seen the value of doing single-leg hops and bounds in our plyometric programs. Why has

Strength and Conditioning Coaching

it taken us so long to embrace single-leg Olympic lifts? I can only say I wish I'd listened to Jeff Oliver 20 years ago.

I'll finish with one more quote: *"When the student is ready, the teacher appears."*

Thanks, Patrice. Thanks, Dan. The student may finally be ready.

Thoughts on Velocity-Based Training

Velocity-based training is rapidly gaining popularity in the strength and conditioning community, and I must admit that at MBSC, we've been slow to adapt to the trend.

There are three main issues.

In the interest of transparency, cost may have been the primary issue that prevented us from at least experimenting with velocity-based training. Most available technology was running at about $1,000 USD per unit. In our situation, this would require a minimum of 14 units and an outlay of $14,000. That's a big obstacle to overcome.

In Wil Fleming's *Velocity-Based Training for Weightlifting*, he recommended a unit from RepOne that was in the $300 range, and we ordered one to experiment with. Vitruve is also producing a unit in the same price range, which we have also experimented with.

Our secondary objection was based on the reliability of some of the commercially available units. At one point, a company that I'll leave unnamed provided us a demo unit. The unit was paired with a phone app and was extremely unreliable. In fact, we had only one staff member who could consistently get it to work.

Our last concern was the most important: Is velocity-based training even a good idea for most athletes? I often use the expression, "good in theory, bad in practice." The idea that we should move weights through the concentric range as fast as possible is exactly that—good in theory, but potentially bad in practice. As I continue to read more about velocity-based training, I see it as poorly taught and misunderstood.

I remember Fred Hatfield in his book *Science of Powerlifting* encouraging what he called "compensatory acceleration." Hatfield's idea was to take advantage of leverage and attempt to accelerate the load as leverage became more favorable. Fortunately or unfortunately, lifts like the squat, deadlift and bench press become easier as we near end range. However, end range is probably where we want to decelerate to prevent injury as we move into joint extension.

I've often said, "Some lifts are done slowly because they're meant to be done slowly." Olympic lifts are intended to be fast. I'm not sure that heavily loaded squats, bench presses and deadlifts fall into the same category. The question with velocity-based training might be "how fast" and avoiding "too slow."

Another flaw I've seen with attempting to move loads faster is that lifters tend to speed up both the eccentric and the concentric phases.

There was a phase when we experimented with sets for time. That was a short-lived experiment for us. I am 100% sure rapid eccentric contraction is a recipe for injury. I also believe that improperly loaded concentric contractions might fall in a similar category.

As a result, we continue to jump, throw and do specific exercises for velocity purposes (Olympic lifts, trap bar jumps, squat jumps), but have yet to fully embrace the idea of velocity-based training.

I will say that as I read more, I understand more. We now have a RepOne and a Vitruve unit and, we continue with small-scale experiments.

CHAPTER 6
STRENGTH TRAINING

Powerlifters are athletes; athletes are not powerlifters.

In the world of strength and conditioning, change comes slowly, and often, not at all. For decades we've blindly done what coaches before us have done, adhering to the party line. As with so many areas of sport and life, change was viewed as a bad idea.

But, as Lee Cockrell said in one of my favorite books, *Creating Magic*:

"What if the way we always did it was wrong?"

For years, coaches simply chased more and more strength—and strength meant the powerlifts or the Olympic lifts. We divided ourselves into tribes, and we fought like tribes. Some were Westside, some were Olympic lifters, some clung to old bodybuilding methods, and we always argued.

Twenty years ago, Mark Verstegen initiated a huge leap. Mark, first at Athletes Performance® and then later at EXOS, proposed the idea that we were performance-enhancement specialists. He pushed us into a new era where we questioned lots of "what we always did."

How Strong is Strong?

Strong at…What?

More Importantly, Is Strong Enough Okay?

The first big question we need to contemplate is, "How strong is strong?"

It's interesting. Ask a strength coach for a good bench press or back squat number for a 200-pound male, and chances are you'll get a quick answer. Everyone may not be in agreement, but everyone will have an opinion.

However, if you ask the same strength coaches what constitutes good single-leg strength or good vertical pulling strength, I don't think you'll get the same level of agreement…or if everyone will even have an answer. The answer might be, "What do you mean?"

If we're going to train for strength, we need to define "strong." Few coaches have, as Vernon Griffith says, "explored the corners," and many coaches are stuck in a conventional mindset. Or maybe just stuck in one corner?

The four-minute mile is a great example of a limiting belief. In 1957, Roger Bannister ran the first four-minute mile. On that day, he broke a 12-year-old record. By the end of that same year, 16 runners had also broken the four-minute mile. It's amazing what people can do once they've seen what's possible. Twelve years to break the record… and 16 followers within a year.

As we've encouraged our larger athletes and female athletes to explore unilateral training and upper-body pulling, we've begun to remove some self-limiting beliefs about strength. Our football linemen can all do chin-ups and single-leg squats. Our female athletes routinely do weighted chin-ups.

The real key to athletic strength is to move beyond the powerlifts or Olympic lifts and move "into the corners."

Total Body Strength

How much strength is enough? That's a question we may need to ask ourselves.

Coaches frequently throw out the idea of a double-bodyweight back squat being a pretty good relative strength indicator, and 20 years ago, I would have tended to agree. However, we no longer back squat, so although this might seem like a reasonable metric for some, my dislike of the exercise makes it useless here.

Over the past 10–15 years, we've adopted the trap bar or hex bar deadlift as being a better indicator of total-body strength. I strongly prefer deadlifts (trap bar only) over squats for a number of reasons.

Fact: Deadlifts involve more muscles than squats. Grip strength and upper-back strength are basically bonus benefits of deadlifts over squats. See Barry Ross's *Underground Secrets of Faster Running* for more on this.

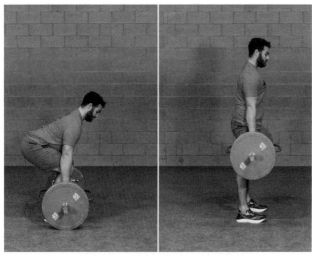

Figure 6.1—Trap bar deadlift, one of our few bilateral strength exercises.

Deadlifts create flexion forces; back squats produce compressive loads. In the deadlift, the lower back must resist a flexion force. The bar is in the hands and the spine is being pulled into flexion. In the squat, the back has to deal with sheer forces and the compressive load of a bar sitting at the cervical-thoracic junction. The sheer force is created by the position of the bar on the shoulders. The bar in the squat is about two feet away from the center of mass, whereas in the deadlift, the bar is more centered.

In addition, torque is a significant issue in squatting. The standard Olympic bar is seven feet long, with plates approximately five feet apart. In the trap bar deadlift, the bar is two feet shorter, with the plates just over three feet apart, creating significantly less torque with similar loads.

The following constitutes "strong" in my experience in some basic exercises for drug-free adult men.

For Men

Bench: 1.25–1.5 times body weight
(250–300 for a 200-pound athlete)

Clean: 1.25–1.5 times body weight (same as above)

Trap bar deadlift: 1.75–2 times body weight
(350-400 at 200 pounds)

Single-leg squat: .5 times body weight for 5 reps
(half of body weight in external load)

Chin-up: .5 times body weight for 1 rep
(half of body weight loaded on a chin/dip belt)

I like athletes to have the same or similar bench and clean numbers. If you don't see this relationship, your athletes are spending too much time benching and not enough time on power movements.

I also like to see the total weight for a chin-up (external load plus body weight) be greater than or equal to the bench press 1RM. In other words, a 280-bench presser who weighs 180 pounds should be able to do one chin-up with 100 pounds.

For Women

Bench: 1 times body weight

Clean: 1 times body weight

Trap bar deadlift: 1.5–1.75 times body weight
(225-265 for a 150-pound athlete)

Single-leg squat: .4 times body weight for 5 reps
(half of body weight in external load)

Chin-up: .3 times body weight for 1 rep
(half of body weight loaded on a chin/dip belt)

As with our male athletes, I also like to see female athletes with the same or similar bench and clean numbers. For them, the total weight for a chin-up (external load, plus body weight) will almost always be greater to or equal to the bench press 1RM. A 150-pound bench presser who weighs 150 pounds will be able to do five to 10 chin-ups, and three to five with 25 pounds of external load.

Another area in which we evaluate strength is by comparing similar or related exercises. It's amazing how many "groove lifters" or specialists we see. Again, in my opinion, strength isn't about how much someone can do in a specialized lift, but the ability to reflect that strength at numerous angles.

With this in mind, we developed the following relationships. Please note: This is in many ways old-fashioned trial and error. Experience over a 10-year period has proven this out.

Bench press = 100%
Example: 300 pounds 1RM

Incline = 80% of bench
or 240 pounds 1RM

Dumbbell incline = 64% of bench press / 2
or 95 pounds 1RM (80 x 5)

Dumbbell overhead = 40–50% of bench / 2
or 60–75 pounds

Overhead pressing is a lost art. It's amazing to see the disparity in overhead pressing strength as it relates to bench press strength. I think most trainees are capable of much more overhead, but no one does it anymore. We still don't push this enough and our athletes don't meet this standard.

We use the following for dumbbell variations.

Dumbbell weight = 80% of bar weight / 2

To continue the 300-pound bench press example:

80% (or 6–7 RM) would be 240 pounds

Dumbbell bench: 6RM would be 80% of 240 / 2 or 95 pounds

A 300–pound bench presser should be able to dumbbell bench 95-pound dumbbells six times.

For incline, we again use the 80% rule. To determine a dumbbell incline 6RM for a 300-pound bench presser, we take 50% of the 1RM divided by two—75 pounds (.8 x .8 x 8 = .51). Another method is to simply take 80% of the flat bench dumbbell weight (.8 x 95 = 76, round to 75).

Our theoretical 300-bencher should be able to dumbbell bench press 95 x 6 and dumbbell incline bench press 75 x 6. If we continue the trend and take 80% of 75, he should also be able to dumbbell overhead press 60 pounds as indicated above—but that's a big "should."

The overhead press is where things fall off. Most athletes in this day and age need a lot of work on overhead movements. Watch most athletes overhead press. They'll make a concerted effort to turn any overhead exercise into an incline press, which allows the clavicular head of the pec to take over for the deltoids in the pressing action.

We now use a progression of half-kneeling overhead press (dumbbell or kettlebell) to standing to force athletes to learn to use the shoulders instead of the chest.

The bottom line for athletes: Strength must exist while standing on one leg and must be demonstrated in more than just a bench press. We're looking for well-rounded strength, not impressive performance on a pet lift. Whenever I have an athlete who arrives as a good bench presser, I immediately shift the focus to the hips and lower body.

I tell my athletes that if they're going to be bad at one lift, I hope it's the bench press. If they're going to be good at just one, I hope it's the hang clean. I'll take hip power over supine strength any day.

A Word About Warming Up in the Weightroom

I was reading Mladen Jovanovic's *Strength Training Manual* the other day, where warm-ups were prescribed by percent of 1RM—50% x 5, 60% x 5, etc.

In a purely theoretical world, this makes sense. In fact, early in my career, I did this with my Excel workout sheets. However, I realized athletes got bogged down trying to get exact numbers on irrelevant sets—not that the warm-up is irrelevant, but whether you do 90 or 95 pounds is irrelevant if your intent is to use 135 pounds.

Teach your athletes to warm up by plates. If I have a strong athlete who's going to bench press 225 x 5, the warm-up is 135 x 5 and 185 x 5. Set one is with 45-pound plates and set two has 45s and 25s. This is simply practical reality.

Be practical; be real. Don't have kids doing math problems during warm-ups.

CHAPTER 7
LOWER-BODY TRAINING

As both a coach and an author, I've taken unpopular stances on lower-body training that have made me both well-known and in many cases, even disliked. About 25 years ago, I came to a conclusion: Athletes I trained would no longer perform the back squat.

As a former powerlifter, I knew this was heresy, but I was tired of a slow parade of athletes making their way to the training room. I found myself constantly coaching our athletes to "keep their heads up" or "use their legs, not their backs," but the pursuit of squat numbers overruled all my coaching. I'd become the master of pounding the square peg into the round hole and had, in the words of Gray Cook, become expert at adding strength to dysfunction.

Much like just about every coach at that time, our emphasis for the back squat was always on increasing weight. This is an American football thing because big squats make football coaches happy. Due to this, squat numbers ruled the weightroom. We tested one-rep maxes two or three times a year and based our success or failure as coaches on these 1RM test outcomes.

The squat poundage increases we so aggressively pursued were often primarily accomplished by altering technique to improve leverage, not by increasing the strength of the muscles so necessary to run or jump. We were inadvertently training powerlifters. We taught wider stances and lower bar carries. We bought better belts. None of these actually made anyone stronger, but the numbers went up.

Teaching powerlifting certainly wasn't the intention, but we were operating under the simplistic notion that more strength would mean more speed and power. And a bigger squat number meant more strength. I still hear coaches quoting stats about double-bodyweight squats and the like, but with no clarification as to what that squat might or should look like.

Our decision to discontinue back squats was based on simple logic that was long overdue. Back squats were responsible for the majority of our athletic back pain, which was ascertained by simple statistical analysis. We looked at the number of athletes with back pain, looked at the reported mechanism, and found the vast majority of back pain complaints came directly as a result of the back squat.

As soon as we eliminated back squats, many "pro-squat" coaches were quick to criticize and point out that we were obviously not good coaches. The rationale was that if we were stricter with technique, back injuries would be avoided. My answer to that defense was always the same—it only took one bad rep to produce a back injury, and in some cases perfect-looking squats were still leading to back pain.

Our solution in the late 1990s was to switch from back squats to front squats. From about 1997 to 2009, our athletes performed only front squats as we continued to pursue bilateral knee-dominant exercises. In 2009, we made another quantum leap when we eliminated the front squat. From 2009 forward, the only heavy bilateral lift we have done is the trap bar deadlift.

Training Hypocrisy

To make matters more confusing, I think everyone should learn to squat. I'm sure I have your head spinning by now. So, you don't have your athletes squat, but you think they all should learn to squat? Let's attempt to clarify.

All beginners, both kids and adults, should become proficient squatters. To us, this means goblet squats done to a low box. What? Double head spin? You just said no box squats and here you're saying to squat to a box?

Just a reminder: This box is a depth gauge, not a spot to sit. We don't sit, we tap.

Does Poor Shoulder Mobility Lead to Low-Back Pain?

I had an epiphany about 10 years ago—you might call it an ah-ha moment. Sometimes when I have these thoughts, I can't decide whether I'm really smart or really dumb. Am I smart because I had this thought or dumb because it took so long?

A member of my staff and I were talking about wall slides. Wall slides are a great exercise we borrowed from physical therapy to develop the combination of shoulder mobility and scapular stability.

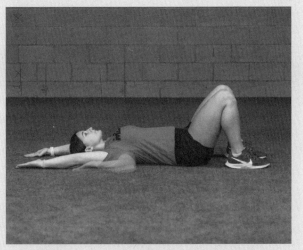

Figure 7.2—Floor slide, a great alternative for a floor-based warm-up.

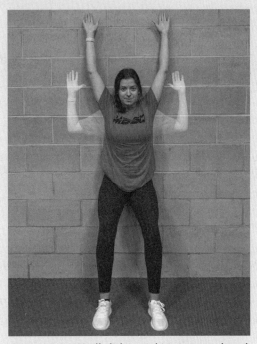

Figure 7.1—Wall slide, working on overhead mobility and scapula stability.

In fact, wall slides and floor slides are two of my favorite upper-body warm-ups and correctives. As the discussion progressed, my young trainer asked about the tendency of our athletes to have to arch their backs to get into a fully externally rotated position to perform the exercise. Strangely, up to that point I hadn't thought about the relationship between shoulder external rotation and lumbar extension.

That's when I realized lumbar extension is the compensation for poor shoulder external rotation. This thought brought shoulder mobility into a new light for me. Poor shoulder mobility suddenly became a major causative factor in back pain—how could I have missed this for so long?

If I try to overhead press and lack shoulder mobility, what do I do? I extend my lumbar spine. If I try to position the bar to back squat while lacking shoulder mobility, I arch my back. If I try to get my elbows up in the clean or front squat and lack shoulder mobility, what do I do? Just like with the wall slide, I extend my lumbar spine.

Similar to how we've realized that the hip and spine are linked, so are the lumbar spine and the shoulder girdle. The next time you have an athlete with low-back pain, don't just look at hip mobility; look at shoulder mobility and at your exercise selection.

This might be why we have less low-back pain when we dumbbell or kettlebell split-squat or when we trap bar deadlift instead of squat. The elimination of forced external rotation in those who lack it may cause a significant decrease in back symptoms. It's amazing what you learn when you stop to listen and think.

Box Squats and Why I Hate Them

Let's start off with a few history lessons. The original Westside Barbell Club was in southern California, where George Frenn and Roger Estep popularized the box squat. In those days, they were often referred to as "rocking box squats," and were done as follows:

"Keeping the hips back, make contact with the butt and much of the hamstrings. For an instant, relax after landing, then rock forward and using this momentum, drive erect."
~ George Frenn

The rock used a bit of momentum to "rocket" the lifter off the bench.

My hatred of the lift probably relates to doing these in the 1970s with over 400 pounds. I still have some consistent back pain 40 years later. It's tough to decide if rocking box squats or maxing in the deadlift every week are to blame, but still, we don't box squat or straight bar deadlift.

I don't care if anyone and everyone does low-load box squats. That's a non-issue for me. When using the term "box squats," I'm envisioning a heavily loaded, power-style back squat. That's the lift I dislike.

Note that there's a distinct difference between "squatting to a box" and "box squats." For the last 20 years, our beginners have done some version of bilateral squats and have squatted to a box to ensure depth. This is totally different than the powerlifting concept of "box squats."

The whole box squat idea has some basic flaws. First off, in the current Westside powerlifting world, the box squat is considered an assistance exercise for the squat. For those of us who train athletes, do we really need to worry about assistance exercises for the powerlifts? We aren't training powerlifters.

Second, I consider the spine to be a fairly delicate structure, prone to problems. Dr. Gunnar Anderson, former chairman of the department of Orthopedics at Rush University Medical Center, states,

"More than 650,000 surgical procedures are performed annually for back pain in the United States with costs exceeding $20 billion. Whether this investment provides good value is largely unknown."

If this is the case, why do we load the spine on top (remember those disc things), and then place something at the bottom (a box)? It just doesn't seem logical. If we look at the core as a cylinder, the best way to crush a cylinder is pressure from the top and bottom, like crushing a can.

If I'm not a back squat fan because I think they're stressful to the back, it stands to reason I'd hate box squats even more.

Another reason I dislike box squats is the pseudo-science that people spout. Louie Simmons from Westside said:

"Every muscle is kept tight while on the box with the exception of the hip flexors. By releasing and then contracting the hip flexors and arching the upper back, you will jump off the box, building tremendous starting strength."

I have no idea how anyone can keep all lower-body muscles tight except their hip flexors and actually relax and contract them while sitting. This seems to be an impossibility in an unloaded situation and insane under load. I also don't see how flexors affect the extensors so necessary to squat. Hip flexors are at best stabilizers in the squat. If someone can explain that to me, I'd be thrilled.

Squatting for Beginners

As I said, we teach every athlete to squat. We've simply chosen a different loading technique. We used to think that before even worrying about back or front squats, every athlete must first learn to bodyweight squat. We've since altered that idea and actually found that a press-out squat or a goblet squat may allow people to learn to squat faster than simply using body weight. For most beginners, we'll use a 10-pound plate to act as a counter balance in the press-out squat.

Teaching an athlete to squat reveals important information about strength, flexibility and injury potential. Squats can be used to assess flexibility or mobility in the hips, ankles and hamstrings, as well as the general strength of the lower body.

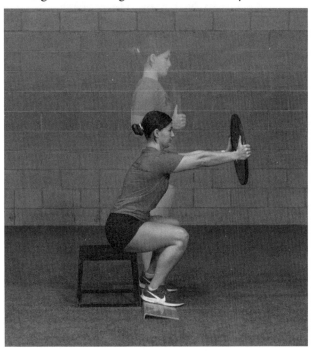

Figure 7.3—Press-out squat, counterbalance is a game-changer.

Elevating the Heels?

On another note, elevating the heels doesn't harm the knees in any way. The idea that elevating the heels increases the stress on the knees isn't supported by any scientific research. In fact, athletes in the sports of powerlifting and Olympic lifting have been wearing shoes with a built-up heel for decades. Lifting shoes were specifically designed to slightly elevate the heel.

People often ask, "Why does elevating the heels help?" The simple answer is that pointing the toes down (heels elevated), opens up more available ankle ROM. The higher the wedge, the more open the ankle and the greater the available ankle range of motion. When athletes run out of ankle ROM either due to a mobility or flexibility limit, the "up-chain" compensations begin.

Why Does the Pelvis Rotate Posteriorly in Some People?

Many coaches describe this as "the butt tucking under" or "butt wink." Coaches see it frequently, but often have difficulty explaining this phenomenon.

To understand better, we need an anatomical explanation. When an athlete squats and maintains a slight anterior pelvic tilt, the hamstrings are actually lengthening during the descent. Athletes with tight lateral hamstrings reach the end of their hamstring range of motion before they reach full squat depth.

As the descent continues and the athlete attempts to get the femur parallel to the floor, the short lateral hamstrings will begin to force the pelvis to rotate posteriorly. Athletes who "tuck under" shouldn't be loaded until they've developed enough flexibility to prevent the posterior rotation. Loading a spine that's moving into flexion is a prescription for disaster. The spine is meant to be loaded in a slightly lordotic position—in an anterior tilt. Loading in a posterior tilt can be dangerous.

Why Do Squats Cause Unusual Inner Thigh Soreness?

As a young coach, I often asked myself that question. Why do athletes often report unusual levels of soreness in an area that appears to be the adductors or the medial hamstrings, and why does it seem even worse with lunges?

I can't tell you the number of athletes I've encountered who described a sensation of "pulling the groin" after being introduced to squatting or lunges. My answer eventually came from Thomas Myers in his book *Anatomy Trains*. Meyers describes the adductor magnus as the "fourth hamstring."

Not only do some people refer to the adductor magnus as the fourth hamstring, but the adductor magnus is, in fact, the third most powerful hip extensor. Many athletes don't use the adductor magnus as a hip extensor until they begin to squat low or perform walking lunges. When they do either of these exercises, they "wake up" the adductor magnus. The response is usually a painful one.

Klaus Wiemann wrote an article called "Relative Activity of Hip and Knee Extensors in Sprinting—Implications for Training." In the article, he describes how the adductor group, primarily the adductor magnus, plays a critical role in sprinting. It acts as both a powerful hip extensor and a counterbalance to the forceful external rotating capability of the glute max. Many in the performance world haven't explored this. In single-leg strength, this fact is even more critical.

ATG and Knees Over Toes

Recently, the idea of below-parallel squatting has gained popularity—dubbed ATG, Ass to Grass or Ass to Ground. The idea of squatting significantly below parallel or deliberately forcing the knees forward over the toes has gained interest from Instagram and around the internet.

I feel the need to tackle both of these topics.

The Squatter's Paradox—Knees Versus Ankles?

Many therapists and athletic trainers like to describe squatting based on a theoretical knee angle. Patients are often directed to squat to a 90-degree knee angle. However, a knee angle of 90 degrees can be attained long before a parallel squat is reached.

Strength coaches, on the other hand, don't define squat depth by knee angle but rather by the relationship of the femur to the floor. A parallel squat can often result in a knee angle greater than 135 degrees if the athlete is an ankle-dominant squatter.

When I wrote the first edition of this book, half-squats and quarter-squats were popular, and we pushed hard to get athletes to squat to parallel. Fast-forward 15 years, and now ultra-deep, below-parallel squats are the trend. Those of us advocating for parallel are perceived as out of date. The pendulum swings and generally swings wildly.

Internet coaches now tout the benefit of below-parallel squatting and encourage athletes to push the knees forward over the toes, seemingly as far as possible.

Coaches debate the entire "knees over toes" concept, and a whole new area of conflict is born.

Knees Over Toes?

It's natural for the ankle to move when squatting, meaning the knee will end up over the toes in a parallel squat. This isn't unsafe for a healthy person.

At MBSC, we don't say, "Don't let your knees go over your toes." However, we also don't say, "Push your knees out over your toes." When you tell someone to push the knees out over the toes, you aren't giving a knee-oriented directive. Instead, you're inadvertently saying, "I want you to use all your available ankle mobility."

We actually cue with phrases like "weight on your heels," "sit back" and maybe even, "lift your toes to the tops of your shoes." In our world, excessive "knees over toes" is a compensatory mistake often used to compensate for poor hip mobility or hip function.

Knees Over Toes and the Patella-Femoral Joint

Recently, I've been exposed to the work of Australian physical therapist Jill Cook. Cook is one of the world's foremost experts on dealing with knee pain, and her number one recommendation for patella-femoral pain is that the exercises must be pain-free.

We've found that "pain free" and super deep, knees over toes squats don't coexist well. In fact, in our experience, it's the opposite. Instead, trying to keep a vertical tibia allows our athletes and clients with knee pain to strengthen pain-free.

The knee joint isn't a simple hinge, even though it may look like one. The patella is the largest sesamoid bone in the body, which acts as a torque converter for the quadriceps mechanism. The patella rides in the trochlear groove and is compressed into the joint in deep squatting.

In addition, the meniscus moves anteriorly as the knee joint flexes, placing the smaller posterior horn in the joint in positions of deep flexion.

Are these positions inherently dangerous? Maybe not. But the big question is what's gained as the person lowers the femur below parallel and pushes the tibia and fibula forward. I've never seen clear medical or injury-prevention benefits linked to these deeper, more extreme ranges. My philosophy is to avoid them.

Goblet Squats to Parallel

As a result, we teach squatting to what's best described as "powerlifting parallel." This means we strive to get the femur parallel to the floor. We neither encourage nor discourage people to get the knees over the toes. Rather, we let nature take its course as we pursue the "right" depth.

We teach beginners the goblet squat to a low box that puts the top of the thighs parallel to the floor. We rarely use partial squats and reserve them for those who experience pain with a deeper range of motion.

In most cases, we don't begin loading athletes until they can do a pain-free parallel squat.

Years ago, partial squats were commonly recommended to "save the knees," but the idea that deep squats are bad for the knees has been debunked. Partial half- or quarter-squats can't fully develop the glutes, hamstrings and lower back.

In addition, half-squats and quarter-squats present a larger risk of back injury due to the heavier weights used in partial movements.

Learning the Goblet Squat

There are two major limiting factors in learning a squatting movement. A lack of hip mobility or a lack of ankle mobility (or both) will often make squatting a challenge.

Another issue can be a lack of understanding of how the hips and the muscles that surround the hips function. The glutes are both extensors and external rotators. As the person descends, the knees should be moving apart. In other words, the hips abduct.

The chest should be up, and the upper and lower back should be slightly arched and tight.

The feet should be slightly wider than shoulder-width apart and turned out approximately 10 to 15 degrees. The stance may be widened a bit to obtain proper depth if flexibility is a problem, but excessively wide stances should be avoided whenever possible.

A one-by-four board, a 10-pound plate or a specially made wedge may be placed under the heels if the athlete tends to lean forward during the descent, if the heels lose contact with the ground or if the pelvis rotates posteriorly in the descent.

Goblet Squat Checklist

Is the movement perfect? If the answer is no, move to step 2.

Add a heel board. Does the squat change? If no, move to step 3.

Plate raise or press-out—I love the plate raise or press-out to create a counter-balance to teach squatting. To do this, you'll have the client grab a 10-pound plate (ideally a large plastic bumper plate), and hold it at hip level. As the person squats down, have him or her raise the plate to head height. My cue is to "Look through the hole in the plate."

Still not perfect? Try putting a band below the knees. The band below the knees teaches new squatters to use the glutes as abductors and external rotators. The band below the knees can be a miracle to someone struggling to learn to squat.

Spanish Squats

Here's another "country" exercise with a name I hate. However, I really like the idea. As mentioned previously, a vertical tibia often allows people with knee pain to squat pain-free.

Key point: the conventionally depicted set-up:

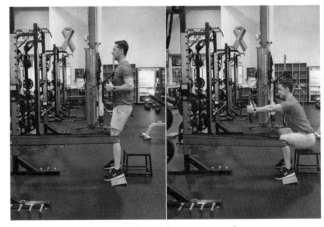

Figure 7.4—Spanish squat, two loops.

This method has the athlete simply looping a band around a rack and placing one leg in each side of the loop. Our set-up is far superior. Instead, we loop the band to the rack first and then both legs go inside the large loop. This allows not only a "sit back" action, but also the addition of abduction and external rotation.

With a Spanish squat, we get a pure knee-dominant movement. As mentioned in the "knees over toes" section, many athletes or clients with patella-femoral pain can't tolerate a knees-over-toes approach. Spanish squats are the literal opposite. The band allows a "sit back" squat that creates a nearly perfect vertical tibia.

If you have clients with patella-femoral issues, try this first.

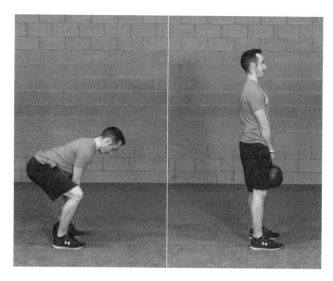

Figure 7.6—Kettlebell deadlift, a great beginner exercise.

Trap Bar Deadlift

The trap bar deadlift, as previously mentioned, has become our major bilateral exercise, replacing both the front and back squats. Trap bar deadlifts are used in our programs for athletes with no history of back pain. Those with a history of back pain don't do bilateral lower-body strength work. Younger athletes begin with a kettlebell deadlift first and progress to a trap bar deadlift.

The bar is always one size, however, and that's a downside. Smaller athletes may end up with a wider grip that makes the lift difficult. This becomes something akin to a snatch-grip deadlift for smaller kids.

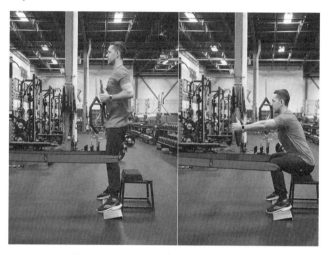

Figure 7.5—Spanish squat, one loop.

Kettlebell Deadlift

The second lift we teach in conjunction with the goblet squat is another bilateral exercise. You're probably thinking, "Gee, these guys do a lot of bilateral training for people who say they don't do bilateral training." Just remember, I consider the main problem with bilateral exercise to be the endless pursuit of numbers.

The kettlebell deadlift should rightfully be dubbed the "kettlebell sumo deadlift." A kettlebell is placed between the feet, with the athlete in a similar setup as the goblet squat. The feet should be slightly wider than shoulder width, and the toes are turned out a bit.

From this position, the person simply squats down to grab the kettlebell handle and rises up. If you think about it, the kettlebell deadlift is probably far more of a squat pattern than a deadlift pattern.

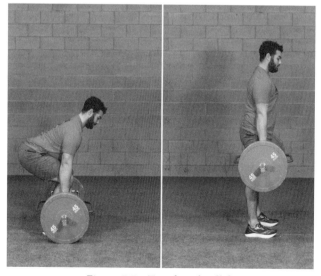

Figure 7.7—Trap bar deadlift.

A trap bar deadlift may be the simplest and most beneficial bilateral exercise we can use. However, there's a great deal of controversy about a squat pattern versus a hinge pattern. Our approach is probably "squattier" than a conventional deadlift.

Learning the Trap Bar Deadlift

Your athlete will stand inside the bar. Use full diameter plates at all times. This means that the lightest weight possible will be 55 pounds—full-size plastic 5-pound plates combined with a 45-pound bar. This creates a proper start position.

Have the lifter squat down to grasp the handles; notice I said "squat." I'm fine with more of a squat pattern as long as the low back stays slightly arched. We tend to use high handles about 80% of the time. This means less ROM and more load. Athletes 5′3″ and under will generally use the lower handle.

Next, tell the person to stand up. Yes, it's that simple. If the load is well selected, it's as simple as standing inside the bar, squatting down to grasp the handles and standing up.

Note: We're "touch and go deadlifters." We don't reset after every rep. I know some coaches feel the "dead" in deadlift means a "dead stop" each rep, but we don't agree. We "tap and go" and try hard not to bounce. The only real key is that the back is slightly arched at all times. The beauty of the trap bar deadlift is its simplicity.

Developing Single-Leg Strength

"All truth passes through three stages. First, it is ridiculed. Second, it is violently opposed. Third, it is accepted as being self-evident."
~ Arthur Schopenhauer, Philosopher

Single-leg strength may be the most important quality in performance training.

When I wrote the first edition of this book, we were clearly in stage one. Over 20 years later, we're very close to stage three! Single-leg strength is a quality that's still ignored or at least undertrained in many strength and conditioning programs. However, it's essential to the improvement of performance, as well as the prevention of injury.

I could make a good case that all bilateral strength exercises are effectively non-functional for most sports. Although eliminating double-leg squatting was once considered extreme, we're seeing more programs either eliminating or de-emphasizing bilateral squatting.

Unfortunately, there are still many strength programs that focus solely on conventional double-leg exercises and even some programs that continue to leg press. Often these same programs also continue to program unequivocally non-functional lower-body exercises like leg extensions and leg curls and attempt make to non-functional exercises "functional" by doing them one leg at a time.

I've said this many times, but ask yourself a simple question: How many sports are played with both feet in contact with the ground at the same time? The answer is close to zero. Almost all sport skills are performed on one leg. For this simple reason, it's critical that single-leg strength be the focal point of a strength program.

Single-leg strength is specific and can't be developed through double-leg exercises. The actions of the pelvic stabilizers are different in a single-leg stance than in a double-leg stance.

Single-leg exercises force the gluteus medius, quadratus lumborum and the adductor group to operate as stabilizers or neutralizers, which are critical in sport skills.

The benefit of single-leg strength development is again reinforced by Weimann's thoughts about the importance of the adductor magnus as both a synergist and stabilizer for the glute max in hip extension. Unilateral exercises force the adductors to act to balance the abduction and external rotation component of the glute max.

Single-Leg Stability or Pure Unilateral Training

The development of single-leg stability is potentially a cure-all for many of the chronic lower-extremity problems we often see in athletes. Numerous athletes suffer from knee problems such as chondromalacia patellae, patellar tendinitis or other patella-femoral syndromes.

Usually, these problems are attributed to problems with the knee joint or patella. Frequently, trainers and therapists describe these problems as patella tracking issues and recommend limited-range strengthening for the quadriceps.

Although this is an outdated concept, many trainers and therapists still cling to these concepts. Sadly, these open-chain non-functional exercises are even making a comeback in the rehab world.

My experience has taught me that most athletes suffering from chronic knee pain generally share a common difficulty in stabilizing the lower extremity while performing a single-leg squat. This inability to stabilize is most frequently a hip dysfunction and isn't actually related to the knee.

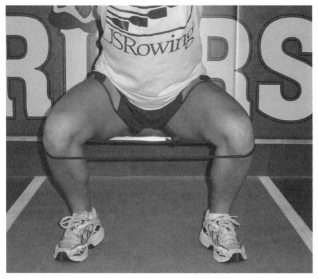

Figure 7.8—Bodyweight squat with a Theratube.

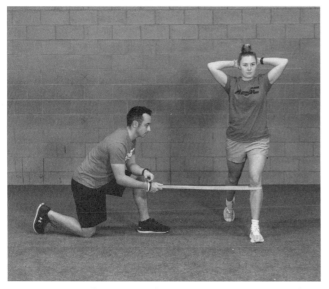

Figure 7.9—Split-squat with RNT, reactive neuromuscular training—basically "pulling into the mistake."

Until recently, many viewed my thoughts on knee pain as related to hip weakness or dysfunction to be my opinion; however, research has validated what was once a hypothesis.

A study by Ireland et. al. validated the hypothesis in an academic setting. Ireland states, "In the absence of sufficient proximal strength, the femur may adduct or internally rotate, further increasing lateral patellar contact pressure. Repetitive activities with this malalignment may eventually lead to retropatellar articular cartilage damage generally associated with this syndrome." [8]

Ireland concluded that healthy subjects had normal strength, while the subjects with patellafemoral pain had significant weakness. Although all subjects in Ireland's study were women, I believe the same results would be seen in men with patellafemoral pain.

Since the early 1990s, physical therapist Gary Gray advocated attacking knee pain from "the hip down," but people in this field are often slow to change. In many athletes, the muscles that control the hip are either too weak to perform their function or aren't properly functioning neurologically. As a result, the support structures of the knees instead of the stabilizers of the hips are forced to provide stability. This may manifest as pain in the iliotibial band, in the patellar tendon or under the kneecap.

In order to better "turn on" the hip stabilizers, a band below the knee joint can be used in double-leg squatting and in some single-leg variations.

The hip stabilizers are often-neglected muscles whose primary function is to stabilize the lower extremity in single-leg movements such as running, jumping or squatting.

Lower-extremity problems were frequently blamed on poor quadriceps strength (or worse, poor patella tracking), and doctors and therapists prescribed simple, non-functional exercises like leg extensions to solve the problem, which, of course, don't work for that.

More recently, therapists and athletic trainers began to recognize the role of the lateral stabilizers in knee problems. Correction may involve facilitation of the hip with bands (is in Gray Cook's reactive neuromuscular training concept, RNT), as well as single-joint isolation exercises to teach athletes how to use and strengthen the hip abductors (from Mark Verstegen's idea of isolation for innervation).

The Ireland work and additional work by Christopher Powers at USC mentioned in the section on single-leg stability are obviously applicable to single-leg strength as well. The work of Ireland and Powers gives additional credence to under-read and under-valued work like Weimann's.

---

[8] *Hip Strength in Females With and Without Patellofemoral Pain*, Mary Lloyd Ireland, MD1 John D. Willson, MSPT2 Bryon T. Ballantyne, PT, MA2 Irene McClay Davis, PT, PhD3 674 J Orthop Sports Phys Ther • Volume 33 • Number 11 • November 2003

Many of our current lower-extremity syndromes could be prevented or alleviated with single-leg training. Single-leg or unilateral training is the logical process of taking what we understand about functional anatomy and applying it to training.

There are muscular differences between double-leg training and single-leg training. The key stabilizers of the pelvis so necessary in any running or jumping activity receive little or no stress in conventional double-leg exercises, and that's my problem with double-leg training.

Single-leg strength is now recognized as a key in injury reduction and has become a staple of most reconditioning programs and knee-injury prevention programs. The next step is to make single-leg training a staple of every strength and conditioning program.

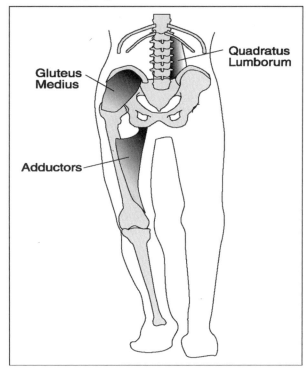

Figure 7.10—Interrelationship of the pelvic stabilizers, courtesy of NASM.

Can Patellas Track?

We still hear doctors and therapists talking about "patella tracking." However, I remember Gary Gray saying 20 years ago that bones don't have nerves or motor function. Bones only go where muscle and connective tissue allow them to go.

The patella can't "track." It's a sesamoid bone contained in the quadriceps tendon. It basically just does "what it's told."

If you think you're looking at a patella tracking issue, you're actually seeing a hip control issue. Think of the hip as the steering mechanism for the knee. Knee control is really hip control.

Valgus collapse is a hip problem, not a knee problem, and a patella tracking issue is really a femoral control issue.

Unilateral Training and the Bilateral Deficit

"What if the way we had always done it was wrong?"
~ **Lee Cockrell,** Creating Magic

Any time we bring long-held beliefs into question, there's bound to be controversy. However, imagine if I said I could show you a new spin on lower-body strength training that would allow you to train with heavier weights and yet was far safer and potentially more effective than what you currently do? I think many intelligent coaches would initially say, "Show me."

Unfortunately, as I began to describe how to lift heavier loads more safely, the sense of what's conventional and acceptable took over. As I began to describe unilateral exercise as a method to use greater loads, the automatic reaction was, "But I'm using less weight."

In truth, you might be using less weight than you'd use in the comparable bilateral lift, but you'd still be using more weight with the targeted muscles. By working only one side at a time, you use what appear to be lighter loads. However, this is primarily a problem of math and secondarily a problem of perception.

As an example, a single-leg straight-leg deadlift using 135 pounds supplies 135 pounds to the involved leg and a load of 135 pounds on the spine. Using 225 pounds in a conventional two-leg Romanian deadlift (yes, I hate the term, but you probably recognize it) places 225 pounds of load on the spinal column, but supplies only 112 pounds of load to the posterior chain of each leg if we assume equal contribution from each leg.

In this example, the targeted muscles are the glutes and hamstrings; the unilateral exercise involves a higher load for the target. The added bonus is a lower load to an area of injury concern—the lumbar spine.

The unilateral exercise provides more posterior-chain load with less low-back stress. Can that be a bad thing? The rational answer is no; however, the reaction is often more emotional than rational.

The next complaint or rationalization revolves around the thought that "the exercise doesn't look like what I'm used to." Unilateral exercises are viewed as weird, different and…*functional*. Unfortunately, I again have to say that's not a good reason not to lift heavier loads, is it?

That these new training ideas "require too much balance" is another frequent complaint about unilateral exercise. This is the most interesting complaint from the free weight community. If I brought up machine-based training, comments like, "Free weights blow away machines," "Machines don't allow you to balance and stabilize the weight," immediately come to mind. In fact, for years we've been told that free weights are superior to machines because we're required to balance the load and are incorporating important underworked stabilizers.

However, when the thought process moves one step further and we ask someone to perform a unilateral exercise, the argument is often reversed.

The unilateral opponent takes the position that unilateral exercises aren't good because they're too unstable and require too much balance. Funny! In one breath, we glorify free weights because of the balance and stability requirements and in the next breath denigrate unilateral training because of the balance and stability needed. This sounds like more of the Simon Sinek lament:

*"Why can't we do what
we have always done?"*

Could it really just be change we dislike?

Do we cling to outdated ideas even in the face of solid evidence?

Henry Ford had a great quote that parallels my position on unilateral training.

*"If I'd listened to my customers,
I would have invented a faster horse."*

If I'd listened to everyone else, we'd still be doing back squats and proclaiming them as the "king of all exercises."

Unilateral training is not accepted because it's different and unconventional. Fortunately (for me) or unfortunately (for nearly everyone else), the evidence is becoming more clear that unilateral training allows for training with higher loads on the targeted muscles.

This brings us to the critical concept of bilateral deficit:

"The bilateral limb deficit (BLD) phenomenon is the difference in maximal or near-maximal force-generating capacity of muscles when they are contracted alone or in combination with the contralateral muscles. A deficit occurs when the summed unilateral force is greater than the bilateral force. The BLD has been observed by a number of researchers in both upper and lower limbs, in isometric and in dynamic contractions. The underlying cause of the deficit remains unknown. One possible explanation is that the deficit occurs due to differences in antagonist muscle coactivation between unilateral and bilateral contractions."[9]

Another potential explanation is much more simple. The brain doesn't like bilateral exercise. Numerous studies have shown that opposite hemispheres of the brain control movement—the right side of the brain controls the left side of the body. This is the natural way the body works. Attempts at simultaneous bilateral contraction is neurologically confusing. The body wants to work one side at a time and does it more efficiently.

The simplest illustration of bilateral deficit can be seen in a hand-grip dynamometer test. The sum of right plus left is greater than the combined score of the two working together. This phenomenon is also seen in leg extension and the single-leg straight-leg deadlift and is also seen in power in the vertical jump/hop (unpublished Boyle data).

The most interesting and useful examples from a strength training perspective can be seen in three exercises. The bilateral deficit is clearly seen in the Olympic lifts (and this drives purists crazy) and in both the rear-foot-elevated split-squat and the previously discussed single-leg straight-leg deadlift. The deficit is so evident in the posterior chain that we've seen greater single-leg straight-leg deadlifts when right and left are combined than in bilateral conventional deadlifts (from Max Shank, a personal conversation and video evidence).

Interestingly, a 1965 study by Bill Kroll showed that the bilateral deficit may be absent

---

9   *Bilateral deficit phenomenon and the role of antagonist muscle activity during maximal isometric knee extensions in young, athletic men. European Journal of Applied Physiol. 2011 Jul;111(7):1533-9. doi: 10.1007/s00421-010-1752-8. Epub 2010 Dec 3. Kuruganti U, Murphy T, Pardy T.*

Strength and Conditioning Coaching

in certain lifts (most notably, in our experience, the bench press), but present in others.[10] Another study showed the bilateral deficit to be greater in some lifts than others.[11]

The bench press example may be explained by the fact that training can actually eliminate the bilateral deficit. With the bench press, the extensive emphasis in many programs may overcome the natural tendency in the body.

In any case, bilateral deficit is real and has been identified and studied since the 1960s. However, in our "why can't we do what we've always done" world of strength and conditioning, we've continually rejected ideas that move us out of our comfort zone.

Coaches like Anatoli Bondarchuck and Frans Bosch laugh at our attempts to copy powerlifters, Olympic lifters and bodybuilders in a quest to create great athletes. European coaches like Bondarchuk and Bosch have emphasized unilateral training for years to improve elite athletes in Europe, but in the US, we're so stuck in the old paradigms that we continue to fight change in the face of science.

If you truly want to improve your athletes, it may be necessary to take a second look at Lee Cockrell's words and ask yourself, "What if the way we have always done it was wrong?"

New Single-Leg Strength Developments

One of the most recent developments in the area of single-leg strength comes again through author David Epstein's "undiscovered connections" idea, courtesy of Australian rules football strength and conditioning coach Alex Natera. Natera et al., in a paper presented at a UKSCA conference in 2015,[12] stated that:

"When comparing or prescribing loads for a single leg squat or jump movements there is a tendency to assume that the load will be half of what the athlete performs in the double leg movement. Whilst this is a reasonable starting point, the reality is that the single leg movement is more challenging, and we can't make that assumption."

Natera used data from a 1955 study on pilot body sizes (for cockpits) and applied it to further our knowledge of single-leg training. The study determined that 68% of body weight is above the hips. Logically, that means unilateral unsupported squatting is at least 16% more difficult than we initially predicted. When we're performing a true single-leg squat, we don't have half body weight—we're using 84% of body weight; 68% above the waist leaves 32% below. Standing on one leg means we have 68% (torso weight), plus the 16% of the free leg for a total of 84%.

To give even more credit where it's due, I have to thank British strength and conditioning coach Daz Drake. His Athletic Performance blog is what led me to Alex Natera's work.

Drake added the following (not in the original UKSCA paper):

BW SL Squat = 1.0 x BW Bilateral Squat

25%BW External loading = 1.5 x BW Bilateral Squat (180 (45))

50%BW External loading = 2.0 x BW Bilateral Squat (180 (90))

100%BW External loading = 3.0 x BW Bilateral Squat

Drake noted that Natera used a Smith machine to maximally load his single-leg squats to a bench, so these numbers might be slightly off.

In any case, we can assume a 160-pound athlete who can perform single-leg squats with 80 pounds of external load (no small task) meets the oft-repeated double-bodyweight squat threshold.

When I wrote *Functional Training for Sports* in 2004, I thought it was great that I had athletes who could do a single-leg squat. I was an early proponent of unilateral training and pushed both my male and female athletes to perform single-leg squats.

In 2007, my thoughts began to change. I noticed a sense of complacency among my athletes. They were just like me—they were happy they could do a single-leg squat with some level of external resistance. Some were actually getting pretty strong, routinely use 20 25-pound dumbbells. Again I initially thought this was great.

---

10   *Central Facilitation in Bilateral versus Unilateral Isometric Contractions, American Journal of Physical Medicine 1965 (44, 218-223).*

11   *Kroll, W Strength-Velocity Relationship and Fatiguabilityof Unilateral vs Bilateral Arm Extension. European Journal of Applied Physiology 1987, 56, 201-205 Vandervoort et al*

12   *https://www.researchgate.net/publication/347623035_LOAD_COMPARISON_RATIO_IN_SINGLE_AND_DOUBLE_LEG_ MOVEMENTS*

Chapter 7—Lower-Body Training

However, they quickly became stagnant. Part of the problem was that over time, the dumbbells became too heavy to properly lift into position and the weight vests we used at the time only went up to 20 pounds. This meant the top weight we were comfortably able to add was about 60 pounds.

The other problem was that we encountered the same issue many coaches encountered in double-leg squats. As the load increases, the depth decreases. To solve the loading problem, we began to use a combination of heavy chains and 40-pound sandtubes.

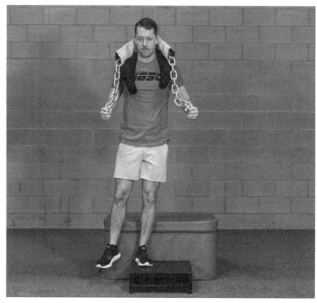

Figure 7.12—Single-leg squat chain plus sandtube—Sandtubes are now commercially available and can be combined with chains.

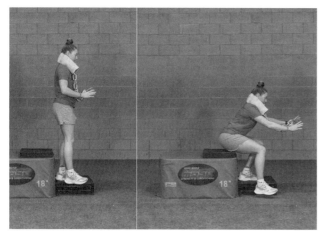

Figure 7.11—Chain-loaded single-leg squat, chains can be an inexpensive weight vest substitute.

To solve the depth problem, we began to use the same method we used to insure depth on our double-leg front squats. We placed a box behind the athletes and asked them to touch it. The only difference was that they were now standing on one leg. Now we could dictate depth and increase load. Sounds like a prescription for success. We were half right.

The "pistol type" version we initially used caused low-back pain in some athletes, particularly those with long femurs. We solved that by using two boxes, one to stand on and one to squat to.

We next actually tested our athletes—testing isn't the same as training. In test situations, athletes compete. The results surprised me. Current Boston University Head Ice Hockey Coach Jay Pandolfo did 95 pounds for 11 reps on each leg. Our Boston University hockey captain did 110 pounds (a 50-pound vest with 30-pound dumbbells) for five reps on each leg. The average for our college hockey team was 80 pounds for five reps.

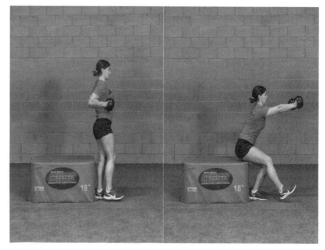

Figure 7.13—Single-leg squat-to-box, use these to teach or reinforce consistent depth. Don't sit, tap.

Now when someone asks me to give them a parameter for single-leg strength, I can tell them that 80 x 5 is good for a single-leg squat and 110 x 5 is excellent. Natera's work took all of this a step further and told us how this related to an actual back squat. This is a huge step, as it aids in the conversion of reluctant bilateral advocates.

As in *Functional Training for Sports*, *Advances in Functional Training* and *New Functional Training for Sports*, single-leg strength exercises are classified as level one, two or three. All athletes generally begin with a level one exercise for the first three weeks of training.

Strength and Conditioning Coaching

Almost all level two exercises can be done with external load by more advanced athletes, but athletes should progress only after they've mastered an exercise.

Most athletes can begin single-leg training with external loads (bar, dumbbells, weight vest…or a combination), but this may be difficult for people who are larger or weaker. Larger (heavier), taller or younger athletes frequently struggle with single-leg exercises in the initial stages.

Resist the temptation to rush into more difficult single-leg exercises if your population includes football linemen, tall basketball players or any athletes with poor leverage or poor strength-to-bodyweight ratio. Almost all young athletes fall into one of these categories.

As athletes become more advanced, you can add any single-leg exercise into the program as long as no fewer than five reps are used.

Is Split-Stance Single-leg?

Recently, some coaches began to argue that split-stance work isn't unilateral. To be truthful, I think this is a bit of a silly semantics argument. I liken the back leg in split-squats and rear-foot-elevated split-squats to an outrigger on a canoe. The existence of an outrigger doesn't make a canoe not a canoe. The outrigger just makes the canoe more stable.

The back foot in split-stance unilateral exercises functions as an outrigger—a stabilizer. The target muscles of the back leg aren't in position to be great contributors, but they do provide stability. In an older article, I categorized these exercises as "single-leg supported" exercises. This was to distinguish between split-position exercises and true single-leg squats. However, the supportive balancing foot doesn't make these exercises bilateral; it only creates some stability for the working leg.

Again, the work of Alex Natera is useful in determining the contribution of the back leg in split-stance exercises. Natera's research indicates that split-squats are 65% front leg, and rear-foot-elevated split-squats are 78% front leg.

Natera's Single-Leg Continuum

Back Squat 50/50 > Split Squat 35/65 >
RFESS 22/78 > Single-Leg Squat 0/100

Level 1—Split-Squat
(65% front leg, 35% rear leg)

The split-squat is the best simple exercise for developing single-leg strength and is almost always step one in our single-leg progression.

In the past, we'd only split-squat for three weeks before moving to a rear-foot-elevated split-squat, but I've changed my thoughts on this. We now attempt to "exhaust" the split-squat before moving to the rear-foot-elevated version.

By exhaust, I mean we continue to use the split-squat until loading becomes an issue. We'll also use a goblet position (one dumbbell end-up, held at chest level) until we "exhaust" our ability to load in the goblet position.

Exhausting the goblet position means we use heavier dumbbells until getting the dumbbell into the goblet position becomes the limiting factor.

At this point, we move to holding dumbbells in both hands.

In the first edition of this book, I advocated barbells in both the front- and back-squat positions. Over the years, we've moved away from barbells for safety reasons. With a bar in the back-squat position, any difficulty could result in dumping a barbell on the extended back leg. This obviously poses a significant danger.

In the front split-squat position, the lifter gets into what's best described as a "bow and arrow" position. The thoracic spine is extended by the bar carry, while the lumbar spine is extended by the rear leg. This may lead to some of the issues back expert Stuart McGill has attributed to unilateral training. In the suitcase position (dumbbell in each hand), we've heard no complaints of lower-back pain.

Performing the Split-Squat

The key to the split-squat is to take a stance that places the back knee just slightly behind the hip. We begin in what Coach Brad Kazmarski calls a "bottom-up" position. This means starting down in a short lunge position with the back knee on a pad. This is to make sure the athlete masters the bottom and middle positions.

If we're loading, we load in the goblet position. Here the cue is "push the head toward the ceiling," pushing through the heel of the front foot.

We tell our athletes to go up and down like an elevator, not back and forth like a saw.

The McGill Split-Squat Controversy (Pelvic Stress?)

Every exercise is a tool to reach a training objective. Proper coaching cues, form and training volume can make an exercise beneficial; yet on the other hand, inappropriate form and volume can lead to musculoskeletal disorders. In recent presentations, Dr. Stuart McGill has expressed concern about the use of the split-squat. We discuss the split-squat in this framework.

McGill: Over the last couple of years, I've seen more patients with pelvic-ring dysfunction. The sacrum posteriorly and the two iliums form the pelvic ring. These bones join one another at the sacroiliac joints in the back and pubic symphysis in the front. The strength athlete needs a tight pelvic ring.

When I review the training history of athletes or patients with low-back and pelvic pain, a number of them were associated with split-squats that were excessive. They used far too much load, far too much depth and excessive volume.

The split-squat, when pushed with longer foot split-stances and when pushed to excessive depth, may cause one ilium to rotate forward and the other side to rotate in the opposite direction. Over time, the SI joints may be stressed to the point of pain, joint laxity and loss in training tolerance.

A case example: A tennis coach realized that lunges are important for tennis, but prescribed far too excessive a depth and volume of split-squats with a barbell on the shoulders. The coach caused the dysfunction—it was a good exercise but using poor technique. Follow the coaching cues outlined by Coach Boyle below to enhance safety and benefit from the split-squat.

Boyle: Split-squat coaching cues to optimize training objectives and minimize poor outcome:

1—We use a relatively short stance. This will reduce torsion in the pelvic ring. A lot of the videos I've seen have the rear leg quite extended. We start just a few degrees past a 90/90 position.

2—We rarely do more than 30 reps per week per leg. A big volume week for us would be three sets of 10 repetitions.

3—We never put the bar in a back- or front-squat position. Positioning the bar this way causes a great deal of lumbar extension, which could increase back and anterior hip stress. We always use dumbbells or kettlebells.

The ATG Split-Squat

The ATG split-squat—the knees-over-toes split-squat—has recently gained popularity on Instagram and YouTube. The emphasis here seems to be that more is better, and the goal seems to be greater dorsiflexion and hip extension. Based on what you just read from Dr. McGill, this may not be a good idea, particularly with heavier loads. In addition, we should be concerned with both potential patella-femoral issues and anterior ankle issues.

Bench-Block Split-Squat

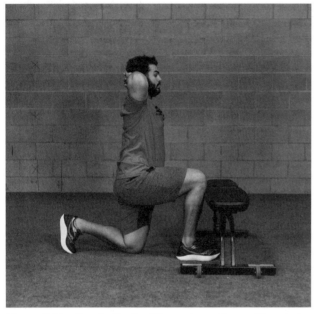

Figure 7.14—Bench-block split-squat, use these with anterior knee pain clients to teach or reinforce a vertical tibia.

A bench-block split-squat is the opposite of the ATG or knees-over-toes split-squat. Our experience has been that many clients with knee pain tend to "saw," which is a large forward weight shift onto the ball of the front foot. In the bench-block split-squat, we use an exercise bench to literally block the anterior weight shift and attempt to maintain the vertical tibia.

By positioning the foot under the bench, we limit the forward translation of the tibia. This changes the knee and ankle angles and reduces patella-femoral joint stress. This often makes the difference between a painful and a non-painful split-squat.

In this case, we're deliberately trying to prevent the knees from going over the toes. As mentioned in the double-leg strength section, knees over toes isn't inherently dangerous, but it can produce or magnify pain in those already suffering knee pain.

We find that the bench-block split-squat can be a game-changer for those rehabbing from ACL reconstruction. Often those who've undergone a patella tendon reconstruction will find knee over toes painful, but knee over ankle pain-free.

Front-Loaded Vertical Tibia Split-Squat

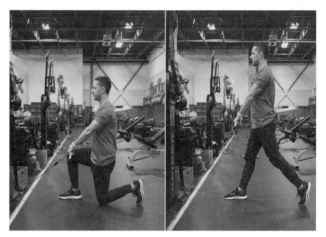

Figure 7.15—Front-loaded vertical tibia split-squat, another great exercise option for those with anterior knee pain.

I know that's a mouthful, but combining a cable front load with a vertical tibia orientation can allow athletes with anterior knee pain to progress pain-free. By loading via a cable system in the front of the athlete, the pushing action is now a "push-back" action. This push-back action decreases the patella-femoral joint loading and creates what we've dubbed "closed-chain terminal extension."

"During backward walking, the rate of patellofemoral joint compressive force loading has found to be significantly lower in later period of stance phase. This reduced rate of loading facilitates the accommodation and prevents the susceptibility to injury of articular cartilage that is rate sensitive to loading due to its viscoelastic properties." [13]

The front-loaded split-squat is another excellent option for someone with patella-femoral pain.

Level 2—Rear-Foot-Elevated Split-Squat (78% front leg, 22% back leg)

The rear-foot-elevated split-squat goes by numerous names. Bulgarian Angel Spassov referred

---

[13] Kedia S, Sharma Saurabh. Effect of retrotreadmill ambulation training in patellofemoral pain patients. *Physiotherapy and Occupational therapy Journal.* 2012; 5(2).

to the exercise as a Spassov squat in the 1980s and questionably attributed many Eastern European successes to its performance. Spassov's promotion of the lift eventually led to the misnomer "Bulgarian lunge." This exercise isn't Bulgarian and isn't a lunge. A lunge involves a step. The term "stationary lunge" is also a misnomer as you can't be stationary and also lunge—you're either stationary or lunging.

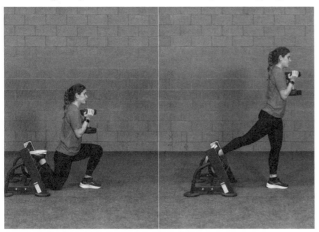

Figure 7.16—Rear-foot-elevated split-squat, neither Bulgarian nor a lunge.

For years, the rear-foot-elevated split-squat has been our go-to unilateral exercise, but that's changing. One thing became apparent as the loads increased: Many athletes just tried to find a way to move the weight. This might best be described as a "back foot, front foot" struggle. Some coaches propose a simple solution and say, "Have them focus more on the front foot," but as loads increase, this becomes more difficult and the lift gets sloppy. For us, this means it's time to move to more emphasis on pure unilateral exercises like single-leg squats and skater squats (which I now view as single-leg versions of the trap bar deadlift).

To perform the rear-foot-elevated split-squat, your athlete will get into a position similar to that for the split-squat, but with the back foot on a bench or one of the newly designed foot stands.

In this position, there's one stable point of support on the floor and one less-stable point on the bench. This is a slight decrease in stability from the split-squat and an increase in difficulty because the back leg can provide less assistance—the back leg contribution drops from 35% to 22%. The exercise is now more difficult as more of the body weight shifts to the front foot and stability is decreased by the back foot position.

From here, have the athlete descend until the front thigh is parallel to the floor and the back knee is nearly touching the floor. We've actually taken to placing an Airex pad under the back knee to provide both a target to touch as well as some cushion.

Like the split-squat, this exercise can improve the dynamic flexibility of the hips while strengthening the legs. The athlete keeps the abdominals tight or additional motion will come from lumbar extension compensation rather than hip motion.

This exercise can be initially done as a bodyweight exercise, following an 8–10–12 bodyweight progression or as a strength exercise with dumbbells. As few as five reps can be used (three sets of five reps per leg). We don't recommend dropping to sets of three as the loads will promote a conflict between the front leg and back leg. Also, my preference is to use dumbbells or kettlebells because dumping the weights is easy. Olympic bars in the front- or back-squat position can create a myriad of problems as the lift becomes heavier and more difficult.

Level 2—Slide Board Lunge (100% front leg)

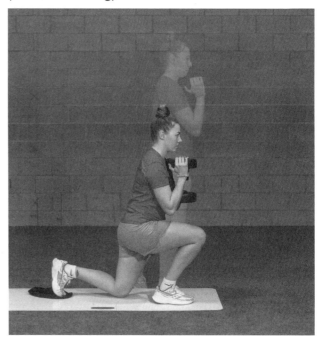

Figure 7.17—Slide board lunge, one of the best and most underused single-leg exercises.

The slide board lunge is rapidly becoming one of our favorite single-leg exercises. In fact, we've now begun to focus on what I call the "Big Four" unilateral exercises: slide board lunge, single-leg squat, single-leg deadlift/skater squat and single-leg straight-leg deadlift with our athletes.

The slide board lunge is an excellent exercise that combines single-leg strength, dynamic flexibility and moderate instability. My affinity for this exercise led me to convince UltraSlide to develop and market a five-foot mini-slide version that's not appropriate for conditioning, but is specifically for exercises like slide board lunges and leg curls.

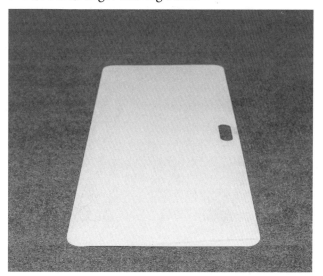

Figure 7.18—Mini-slide board, a great space-saver that allows lunges and leg curls to be done anywhere.

One of the unique benefits of the slide board back lunge is that it's a hip-dominant exercise that looks like a knee-dominant exercise. Slide board lunges can train the posterior chain with very little spinal stress.

Craig Freidman from EXOS maintains that the movement pattern of the front leg is more of a pulling action as the sliding foot moves forward. This pulling action stresses the hip extensors to a greater degree than the knee extensors. In *Functional Training for Sports*, I classified these exercises as hybrids, exercises that seemed to be a combination of knee and hip dominance.

Slide board lunges are probably best started by using a bodyweight progression (body weight x 8–10–12) because of the additional stretch and instability component. However, the reason we include these in the Big Four is because they're a "cheat proof" strength exercise when done properly. Our goal in this particular exercise is to hit Natera's target of 50% body weight relatively quickly.

Beginners move from body weight to goblet loading to suitcase loading. This is another exercise where we ideally want to "exhaust" goblet loading before moving to the suitcase position.

Level 3—Single-Leg Squat
(100% working leg, 84% of body weight unloaded, 50% of body weight in external load = 2 x bodyweight squat)

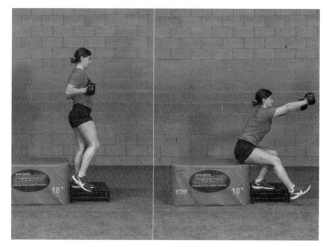

Figure 7.19—Single-leg squat, the real king of lower-body exercises.

The single-leg squat is another of the Big Four and in my mind is the king of single-leg exercises. We categorize these as "unsupported single-leg squats" because the support of the back leg is now completely eliminated. It's probably the most difficult and also the most beneficial of all the single-leg exercises—although I could also make a case for the single-leg deadlift.

The single-leg squat requires the use of one leg without any contribution to balance or stability from the opposite leg. The pelvic muscles must function as stabilizers without the benefit of the opposite leg touching the ground or contact with a bench, stand or another surface.

I can't overstate the importance of this point because pelvic stabilization is critical in all sprinting actions. In sprinting, the stance leg must produce force without assistance from the swing leg.

Don't get discouraged if your athletes initially struggle to perform this exercise. Most people feel unsteady or clumsy the first few times. Even good athletes might require a few sessions to become comfortable with a true single-leg squat.

A Pistol Is a Single-Leg Squat, but a Single-Leg Squat is NOT a Pistol

Don't confuse single-leg squats with pistol squats.

Let me be very clear: We neither do nor endorse pistol squats. Although these two exercises may seem similar, they aren't interchangeable in name or performance.

With a single-leg squat, there's significantly less stress on the hip flexors, and subsequently less stress on the lower back than in a pistol squat. In the single-leg squat, the non-working leg isn't required to be parallel to the floor, and various set-up options can be used. This decreases the use of the hip flexors and decreases the potential for back pain.

A pistol squat is generally done standing on the floor and, in my opinion, can be more of a circus trick than an exercise. Have you noticed how people love to be able to show you they can do a pistol? I must admit, being able to do a pistol is a nice party trick, but in my mind, it isn't great training.

Here's the fundamental difference. Performing a single-leg squat without the requirement of holding the free leg parallel to the floor drastically changes the exercise.

Standing on a box may be the least stressful set-up position for the back, as it allows the free leg to fall to any angle, even potentially perpendicular to the floor.

In a single-leg squat to a bench or box, the free leg can generally be held at about a 45-degree angle to the floor versus the parallel-to-the-floor relationship necessary for a pistol.

Because of the position of the non-squatting leg, pistol squats can often cause low-back pain due to overuse of the hip flexors. Holding the free leg extended and parallel to the floor can produce significant low-back stress and subsequent low-back pain, particularly in people with longer legs. In addition, there's no added benefit provided to the working leg from holding the non-working leg parallel to the floor.

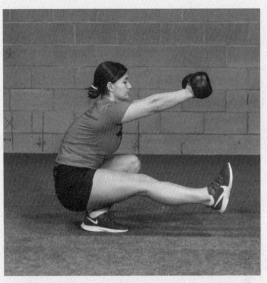

Figure 7.20—Pistol squat, a great party trick and a great way to get a sore back.

Our version of the single-leg squat is most often done to a femur-parallel position. No attempt is made to go below parallel. Below-parallel squatting often results in lumbar rounding. Although this may not be particularly dangerous with no load, it can be a potential problem as the load increases. In addition, below-parallel squatting may cause the posterior aspects of the medial meniscus to be compressed in the joint line. During flexion of the knee, the meniscus moves forward in the joint. In below-parallel squatting, the posterior aspect of the meniscus (the posterior horn) can be "pinched" in the back of the joint.

Bottom line, I love single-leg squats, but I don't even like pistols.

Learning to Single-Leg Squat

Counterbalance

We generally start teaching athletes to perform single-leg squats by holding five-pound dumbbells or plates in their hands. This may be one of only two cases of an exercise being easier with weight than without, a press-out bilateral squat being the other. The counterbalance keeps the body weight back toward the heel. Strangely, five pounds in each hand helps make the exercise easier, but 10 pounds in each hand increases the difficulty.

Other methods to increase resistance for stronger athletes are to combine a weight vest or chain with dumbbells or to use sandbags in the Zercher position. Sandbag Zercher single-leg squats have become the preferred method for our stronger athletes. Some stronger athletes find they're limited by their ability to lift the dumbbells to shoulder height as they increase weight. The Sandbag Roll from Perform Better is another nice development. These are more comfortable than chains as the load increases and can be combined with the sandbag.

We've had larger athletes use up to 25-pound dumbbells, but shoulder fatigue becomes an issue. If the formula calls for 70 pounds, a 20-pound vest can be combined with 25-pound dumbbells or a 40-pound sand collar can be used with a 30-pound sandbag.

Facilitating the Hip Stabilizers With Cross-Body Reaching

If an athlete seems to have the leg strength to perform a single-leg squat but struggles with stability, you can use what we call a "cross-body reach." These athletes may easily perform a single-leg squat, but are unable to keep the knee from moving into an adducted position. Although some might describe this as the knee "falling in" or "caving in," this is actually a hip issue, specifically a glute issue. In many cases, simply facilitating the glutes will solve the problem.

The question is how. In the past, we found ourselves trying to verbally instruct athletes to "not let the knee fall in." This often appeared to be a waste of time because people are often unable to make the connection between the instruction and the action.

Our current solution is to increase the glute max contribution by recognizing that glute max is both an external rotator as well as an extensor. Our instruction for athletes whose knees "cave in" is to *reach across the working leg* rather than reaching straight outward.

This reaching action rotates the pelvis against the femur and increases the contribution of the glute, as the glute is now asked to externally rotate the pelvis on the femur, as well as create hip extension.

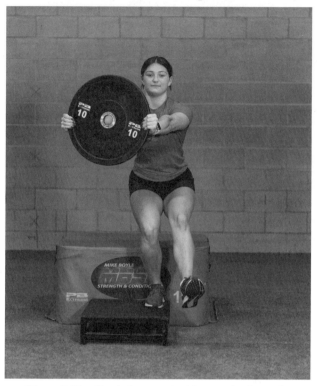

Figure 7.21—Single-leg squat with cross-body reach, reaching across the body rotates the pelvis on the femur and recruits the glutes.

Heel Lifts for Single-Leg Squats?

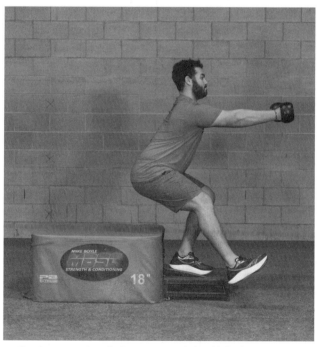

Figure 7.22—Single-leg squat with heel lift (foot on box), a great way to "clean up" a single-leg squat.

I'm often embarrassed to admit my slow uptake on ideas. For years, we've used squat wedges to help us "clean up" our bilateral squats, as discussed in the section on squatting. It took us a while to realize we could cut these to six inches and use them for single-leg squats. For many of our athletes and clients, the single-leg squat "mini wedge" is a quick game-changer.

Lunges Versus Walking Lunges

Lunges are an interesting single-leg exercise category. I'd put conventional lunges in the "decelerative" category and walking lunges in the same category as slide board lunges, viewing them as a pulling exercise.

With a conventional lunge, there's a step forward, a stop and then a pushing back action. This is a decelerative action stopping forward momentum. Conventional lunges are anterior-chain dominant and are great for training braking action. In all honesty, conventional lunges are one of the best exercises we don't use enough. As I sit and write, I think, "We need to get these into the program more."

Walking lunges are really just a moving version of the previously described slide board lunge. It's my belief they aren't used by more coaches due to space issues than for any other reason. The need for a way to load and room to walk make walking lunges impractical in many gym settings. The advent of the portable mini-slide board allows us to gain the benefits of walking lunges in a limited space via slide board lunges.

Step-Ups, Step-Downs and Single-Leg Squats

There's a lot of confusion in the fields of strength and conditioning and physical therapy about naming and using single-leg exercises. I often see the terms "step-up," "step-down" and "single-leg squat" used interchangeably. Many coaches find these three exercises similar; they share similar movement patterns, yet they're distinctly different.

Step-up *(50% BW up leg)*—It seems that step-ups would fall in the 82% front-leg category, but research shows that most people push off the floor with the down leg, as well as into or down on the box with the up leg. This makes the step-up a potentially good exercise for beginners.

However, step-ups aren't always a great choice as a strength exercise for the same reason…but oddly, they remain popular. I think it's because they're an easy exercise to cheat on. This is what makes them good for beginners and potentially not-so-good for more advanced athletes.

For most people, step-ups are a true combination exercise. They're usually a combination of the extensors of the working leg and the calf of the non-working leg. The bottom line for me is that step-ups are hard to do well and easy to do poorly. That makes them a poor choice for anyone except beginners.

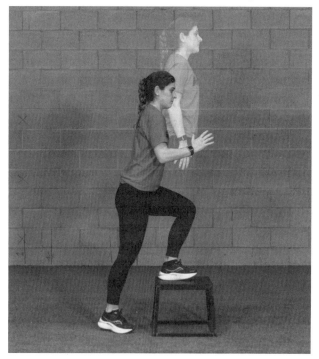

Figure 7.23—Step-up, a great general population starter exercise.

In addition, step-ups have another huge drawback. A step-up begins with an almost pure concentric contraction. In that way, they're similar to chin-ups. For athletes with knee problems, particularly patella-femoral issues, step-ups can be an uncomfortable exercise that can cause or magnify knee problems. Without the preceding eccentric component found in most squatting exercises (starting in extension loaded by gravity), there's knee discomfort that could otherwise be avoided.

Often athletes with patella-femoral pain find single-leg squats or step-downs relatively comfortable, but experience pain with step-ups. This makes sense, as step-ups begin in knee flexion with little-to-no preceding eccentric load. Imagine asking someone with bad shoulders to bench press off the pins of a power rack. I think anyone with shoulder issues will cringe. There's a clear benefit to eccentric preloads when it comes to the patella-femoral joint—and probably the shoulder joint.

In spite of the negatives, step-ups can be a great explosive exercise for athletes with healthy knees. In fact, explosive step-ups are my favorite exercise in any knee-dominant complex or contrast sequence.

Step-down—a step-down isn't actually a step down at all; it's a limited range single-leg squat.

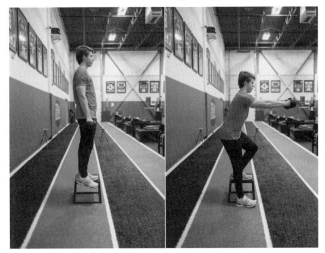

Figure 7.24—A step-down is really a single-leg squat off a 12-inch box. This is another example of the poor terminology we're often saddled with in our field. A better name would be a "lower down." I like step-downs as a progression to a single-leg squat. I just don't like the name.

The key difference between a step-down and a step-up is that the step-down begins with an eccentric contraction. The major difference between step-downs and single-leg squats is that step-downs are intentionally a limited range exercise designed for rehab or are used for weaker athletes who can't yet single-leg squat. By contrast, a step-up is a concentric action of hip and knee extension with relatively no preceding eccentric contraction.

The key to the step-down is to never lose the eccentric load. In step-downs, the free leg often goes behind or to the side, but is held relatively straight.

In a step-down, the concentric action is in effect "set up" by a preceding eccentric contraction. The key to patella-femoral health may be that the preceding eccentric contraction allows the patella to sit properly in the trochlear groove.

A step-down is most often done from a low box, usually 12 inches, to a heel or toe touch. It's an excellent way to begin to develop both lower-body strength and femoral control, but it is really a deliberately range-limited single-leg squat.

Single-leg squat—the single-leg squat is the king of single-leg exercises and the gold standard in rehab. In a single-leg squat, the body is now unsupported and the range can be as large as tolerated. Ideally, athletes can single-leg squat to a position where the femur is parallel to the floor. Unlike the step-down, in the single-leg squat, the free leg is carried slightly in front and never touches the floor.

In the pistol-type single-leg squat that I'm not a fan of, the free leg is held out in a parallel position and the spine is allowed to go into a posterior tilt. We've had problems with back spasms and hip flexor cramps when we attempted this lift, particularly with taller athletes.

The effort needed from the rectus femoris, psoas and iliacus can cause problems in the low back. For this reason, we advocate that the free leg is held just high enough to clear the floor and there's a more deliberate attempt to maintain a flat lumbar spine. We also always use at least five pounds in each hand to create counterbalance. This allows a flatter back by encouraging thoracic extension and eliminates the large posterior tilt of the pistol single-leg squat.

Considering the Differences

These exercises, although seemingly similar, have significant differentiating points. Think of step-ups as an exercise to be used sparingly and by healthy beginners. Think of the step-down as a rehab progression toward a single-leg squat. The step-down is really just a controlled short-range single-leg squat.

Hip-Dominant Exercises

A chapter on hip-dominant exercise could actually be an extension of the core chapter, or it could follow the knee-dominant exercises as it does here. When does an exercise like bridging cease to be an exercise for core stability or glute activation and become a strengthening exercise for the hip extensors? In reality, the line between a core exercise and many hip-dominant exercises is almost impossible to draw.

Many of our core stabilization exercises are actually foundational movements that become the basis of proper execution of our hip extension exercises. The concept of glute activation and utilization learned from the bridging exercises directly carries over and into all of our bent-leg hip-extension exercises and Nordic variations. The bent-leg hip-extension exercises like hip lifts and leg curls are simply progressions from bridging, adding a concentric/eccentric emphasis.

The training of the entire posterior chain, as the glute and hamstring group are often referred to, becomes more vital as we begin to further our understanding of functional anatomy. The posterior chain works in conjunction with the quadriceps to control all locomotor movement, from walking to running.

Janda referred to the systems of the posterior chain as the "deep longitudinal subsystem" and the "posterior oblique subsystem" and demonstrated how critical these muscles are in transferring force from the ground to the upper body.

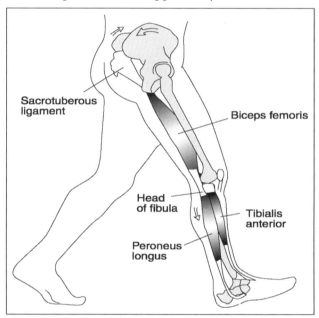

Figure 7.25—The deep longitudinal and posterior oblique subsystems.

When the foot hits the ground, the ankle is stabilized by the tibialis anterior and peroneals. This allows force to be transmitted through the hamstrings into the glute max. If we don't perform single-leg hip-extension exercises, we'll again miss a critical part of both force transmission from the ground and ankle stability.

Standing hip-dominant exercises must begin at the ground with the peroneal group and tibialis anterior, and then proceed literally up the chain through the lateral hamstrings and into the glutes.

The use of the thoracolumbar fascia as the crossing point through the lumbar spine reinforces our core training concepts as both the transverse abdominus and internal oblique act on the same thoracolumbar fascia.

Movement is linked from the feet to the shoulders by the core muscles and fascia.

Unfortunately, the muscles that extend the hip, primarily the gluteus maximus and hamstring group, are often neglected in many training programs. When we view the systems from a functional anatomical perspective, it's obvious that hip-dominant exercise is as important or potentially more important than knee-dominant exercise. Yet many coaches mistakenly believe that squatting is enough exercise for the entire lower body.

Amazingly, some programs are still characterized by a "leg day" that consists mostly of squat-type movements with a token hamstring exercise thrown in. Although I'd love to believe that prone single-joint leg curls have become extinct, I'm confronted frequently with evidence to the contrary. These outdated programs place excessive emphasis on the knee extensors and neglect the hip extensors. This leads to the ever-present possibility of a hamstring strain.

In the 1990s, the Olympic lifting community popularized the Romanian deadlift, and for many coaches the "RDL" is the hamstring exercise of choice. This deadlift is basically a hip hinge done with a limited knee bend. The movement became popular after Romanian Dragomir Ciroslan became the coach of the US weightlifters.

Interestingly, many US powerlifters used this lift for years prior to the introduction of the term "Romanian deadlift." Some did them with a flat back similar to what we know as the Romanian deadlift. Others did them in a round-back style, often off blocks.

In either case, we've abandoned all bilateral hip-hinge variations and use only unilateral choices. In fact, for more than 30 years, we haven't done any Romanian or straight-leg bilateral deadlifts.

In recent years, "hinging" has been re-popularized. People spent all day teaching how to hinge properly, citing the fundamental nature of the movement. I'd like to ask a simple question: Why do they think hinging is fundamental? What skill or skills are enhanced by the ability to forward bend with both legs slightly bent? We're constantly cautioned to bend our knees when picking things up to avoid a "hinge" type of pick up.

Ask yourself, "When does a bilateral hinge really happen?" My thought is never. Or maybe…rarely.

If you study the subsystems discussed in the single-leg strength section, it becomes obvious that unilateral exercise is critical to the proper function of both the anterior and posterior chains.

Although some anatomy texts still describe the hamstring group as knee flexors, science now tells us the hamstrings are actually the second most-powerful hip extensor, as well as being critical stabilizers of the knee and pelvis. Although hamstrings may function as knee flexors in non-functional settings in any locomotor activity, the function of the hamstring group isn't to flex the knee, but to assist in extending the hip. As we shift from walking to sprinting, the hamstrings take on an isometric/eccentric role to control and limit leg extension.

As we better understand functional anatomy, it becomes obvious why exercises like lying or standing leg curls are a waste of time for athletes. Standing or prone leg curls train the muscles in a pattern rarely used in sports or even in life. The outdated process of training and then retraining the hamstring muscles in non-functional patterns may explain the frequent recurrence of hamstring strains in athletes who rehabilitate with exercises such as leg curls or through the use of seated isokinetic machines such as that made by Cybex.

More importantly, strengthening the hamstrings in the absence of proper glute function is simply attempting to train a synergist to do the job of a prime mover. Most hamstring injuries are actually the result of poor glute function and strength. If the glutes function poorly, the hamstrings becomes what Janda calls "synergistically dominant." In other words, we have a synergist attempting to perform the task of a weak prime mover. Over time, the hamstrings will tire and eventually strain.

If the solution to a hamstring strain is more hamstring strengthening, as is often the case, the cycle will continue. As a coach or therapist, when you see a hamstring strain, look for a weak glute. Sahrmann's quote from the earlier pillar strength section bears repeating in this context:

"When assessing the factors that contribute to an overuse syndrome, one of the rules is to determine whether one or more of the synergists of the strained muscle is also weak.

When the synergist is weak, the muscle strain is probably the result of excessive demands."

It's now become our habit to look for a weakness causing the strain, and then to strengthen the weak muscle as well as the strained muscle. This may explain the frequent complaint by athletic trainers and therapists that, "I can't believe he pulled his hamstring again; he had great strength." But in many cases, hamstring weakness was never the primary problem. Instead, the problem was a weak prime mover.

Exercises like slide board or stability ball leg curls are exceptions to the "no single-joint exercise" rule. These types of leg curls use a closed-chain movement where the foot is in contact with a supporting surface, and require that the glutes are isometrically active to maintain hip extension.

How We Currently Train the Posterior Chain

We've got Nordics, Bosch Isos, Razors, the NordBord, glute hams, hip thrusts, reverse hypers, sprints…and the list goes on.

When I wrote the first edition of this book, I was simply trying to get coaches and athletes to:

Get away from non-functional leg curl variations

Move away from quad-oriented, squat-centered workouts

Now we have more information to build upon.

What's the best way to prevent hamstring injury?

How can we best train the posterior chain?

What works best?

What's most functional? What's the least functional?

Let's start with least functional. In my mind, any type of leg curl machine is still the least effective functional hamstring exercise. We haven't done anything like these for 20 years.

Whether lying, seated or standing, attempting to use the hamstrings without some type of simultaneous glute involvement is at a minimum a waste of time from an injury prevention standpoint.

The Shirley Sahrmann concept of "any time a muscle is injured, look for a weak synergist" supports the theory that hamstrings get injured when glutes are weak. Logically, strengthening the hamstrings in isolation seems to make little sense from an injury prevention standpoint. Exercises like slide board leg curls can be used to develop the hamstrings in concert with the glutes.

What's the most functional posterior-chain exercise? A well-designed short sprint program might be the most functional injury prevention tool we can do. Notice three key words, "well designed" and "short."

Tim Gabbett's research has shown that distance matters. Tony Holler's work has shown that volume matters, and JB Morin's work has actually described sprinting as a "vaccine" against hamstring strain.

To further stir the pot, Frans Bosch's work called into question the actual function of the hamstrings in sprinting, and this resulted in an increased interest in hamstring isometrics. "Bosch Iso's" of varying types have become quite popular, and his idea of the hamstrings as more of an isometric brake than an eccentric control mechanism is a concept to consider. (Note: the difference between Bosch's muscle slack idea and an eccentric contraction may be small and of limited practical training consequence.)

Bosch's work is somewhat in contrast to the "Nordic" idea that has also become popular. Nordics (another name I hate) are an interesting subcategory and seem to be surrounded by some confusion. In reality, these are just a better marketed version of Dr. Michael Yessis's glute-ham raise. The positive aspect of Nordics is that some versions don't require equipment. These can be done with a partner or by securing the heels under something like a dumbbell rack.

Unfortunately, there are two big negatives to these Nordics.

One, they're generally too difficult for most athletes and as a result, are generally performed poorly. Ninety-nine percent of the YouTube videos I've seen of Nordic-type exercises are poorly done, generally as a result of poor control of the lumbo-pelvic segment.

Second, the eccentric emphasis can produce extreme soreness.

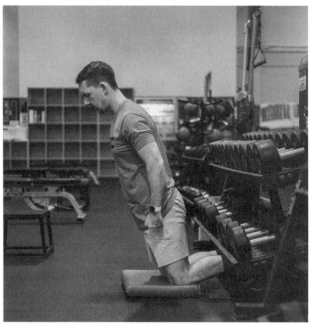

Figure 7.26—Nordic iso start (heels under rack)—the big mistake with Nordic variations is eccentric before isometric!

A note about soreness: In the athletic world, soreness is a no-no. Athletes hate to be sore, especially in-season. Sadly, most modern athletic seasons last six to nine months, so soreness is something to be avoided rather than pursued.

One thing is true: When athletes can actually do both the eccentric and concentric portions of a true Nordic leg curl or glute-ham raise with good lumbo-pelvic position, they have extremely strong hamstrings and probably a lower chance of injury.

The fascination with Nordics and hamstring injury in the international soccer community led to the development of the NordBord, an extremely expensive proposed solution to the problem of hamstring injury. Although the NordBord may be a reasonable idea, it's out of the reach of most athletic programs, so we won't consider it here. In fact, the cost of one NordBord could outfit a small team facility.

Much like Nordics, glute-ham raises are poorly understood and most often, poorly performed. The general downside of the glute-ham raise is the need for some type of specialized equipment. Personally, I'm a fan of the small, lightweight portable glute-ham pads, but even these have their drawbacks. But an athlete who can properly do a glute-ham raise will generally have good hamstring strength and again, a lower chance of injury.

My personal favorite posterior-chain exercise is the single-leg straight-leg deadlift.

The single-leg straight-leg deadlift uses both the glutes and hamstrings as hip extensors and can be heavily loaded after some practice. Many still refer to this as a single-leg Romanian deadlift, but as previously mentioned, I refuse to use names like Romanian deadlift, Bulgarian split-squat, Nordic leg curl or Copenhagen adductor.

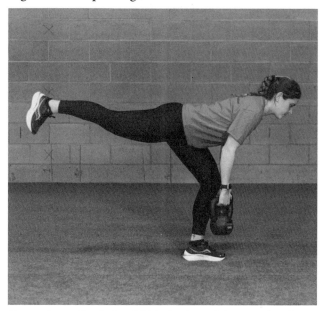

Figure 7.27—Single-leg SLDL, the king of the posterior chain.

Recently, I've begun to view sled pushes as a functional posterior-chain strength exercise.

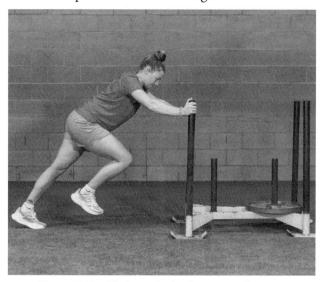

Figure 7.28—Sled march, think reps, not distance.

In the past, sled pushes were somewhat randomly used in the "work capacity" category. In the summer of 2018, we moved sled pushing into our strength program and began to treat sled pushes as a type of horizontal push exercise. Charlie Francis discussed this in his book and used the old Universal Gym leg press for a sort of posterior-chain leg press. In our case, the sled push fills the same bucket.

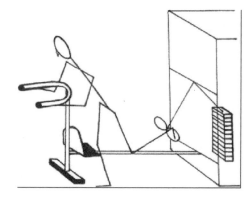

Figure 7.29—Charlie Francis reverse leg press.

The hip thrust is another posterior-chain exercise that's become internet and Instagram popular. I'm not a hip thrust fan for a number of reasons, mainly:

> *Most of the demos I see lack lumbar control and are more lumbar extension than hip extension.*
>
> *Hip thrusts are heavy and bilateral and not entirely comfortable, even with a thick pad. When I think, "heavy, bilateral and uncomfortable," it becomes a tough bandwagon to hop on.*

However, I do like the unilateral version of the hip thrust. We've found that chains work well for resistance. Another great option is the new Sandbag Roll from Perform Better.

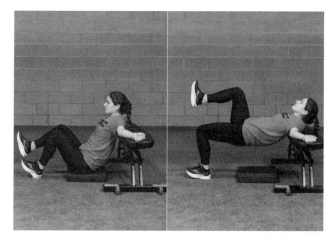

Figure 7.30—Shoulders on the bench hip lift, a unilateral improvement on the hip thrust idea.

To increase the comfort of heavy chains, we managed to find some old "retired" fire hose. We cut two-foot lengths and drop the chain into the hose.

The last piece of the puzzle and the biggest innovation in hamstring training may be the use of timed sprints. Sprinting for time may be the most functional approach to hamstring training and subsequent injury prevention. As previously mentioned, JB Morin proposed the idea of "sprinting as a vaccine" in his article of the same title. Morin's theory is that nothing may be more functional, specific and preventative than the actual act of sprinting.

The high-speed sprinting that many coaches (I'm included) previously avoided out of fear of injury may in fact be a form of mithridatism.

What the Heck Is Mithridatism?

Wikipedia- "Mithridatism is the practice of protecting oneself against a poison by gradually self-administering non-lethal amounts. The word is derived from Mithridates VI, the King of Pontus, who so feared being poisoned that he regularly ingested small doses, aiming to develop immunity."

Yes, short timed sprints may in fact be the non-lethal doses we need to prevent hamstring injury caused by an ill-timed maximal sprint.

The idea of timed sprinting, combined with a Tony Holler approach of timing and recording times weekly, might be the best hamstring injury prevention strategy we can do. We'll get into more detail in the speed development chapter.

We've taken to timing 10-yard sprints twice per week, beginning with a Flying 10 with a five-yard fly-in (15 yards total) and then a Flying 10 with a 10-yard fly-in (20 yards total). We work up to 30 yards (20-yard fly-in, 10-yard timed Flying 10).

We generally time twice each week, performing two or three reps per day, four to six per week. The result for us has been no hamstring pulls and remarkable speed increases. Short sprints might just be the best preventative bang for the buck, as sprints will both prevent injury and enhance performance.

Sprinting has also changed my view of velocity-based training. With bad sprinters moving eight yards per second and good ones moving more than 10, it seems silly to be worrying about weightroom stuff that's under two meters per second.

In the big picture, the best overall prevention strategy might be a strength program that incorporates concentric exercises like the single-leg straight-leg deadlift, isometrics a la Bosch, eccentric emphasis (think Nordic lowers or eccentric slide board leg curls) and a regular dose of timed sprints.

So, the real answer is that there's no single answer. As usual, the best option is a recipe of the right items in the right amounts, rather than picking a few items off a menu.

The best prevention program takes pieces of each concept and weaves them together into a strong protective blanket.

Important Notes

Core control matters—The best way to screw up hamstring training is to elicit hamstring contractions without glute contraction and anterior core control.

In order for any of the many hamstring exercises to be effective, the pelvis must be properly positioned. Athletes must learn to stabilize the lumbar spine before they can truly benefit from hamstring exercises like Bosch isos, Nordics or glute-hams. Many of the internet videos of athletes performing these exercises completely miss this major point. An understanding of the basics of bridging must precede all of this.

Sets and reps—With isometrics and eccentrics, I like to keep the sets and reps low. For isometric hamstrings, we might start with three five-second holds, adding an additional five-second hold each week over a three-week period. For eccentrics, we might use five-second lowers with two or three reps and two or three sets.

Hip-Extension Hamstring Exercises

Hip-extension exercises split into two distinct movement patterns: straight leg and bent leg. It's essential to use movements from both categories to properly train the posterior-chain muscles.

Although some experts claim that bent-leg hip extension isolates the glutes, I haven't found this to be true for closed-chain movements. When the foot is in contact with a surface (stability ball, ground, slide board top), both the glutes and hamstrings work to some degree. Depending on the starting length of the hamstring group, the hamstrings will emerge as either the prime mover or the synergist.

Both straight-leg hip extension and bent-leg hip extension target the glute and hamstrings. The difference lies in the concept of length-tension relationships. Length tension basically dictates that muscles will work best at normal length. If they're shortened or overstretched, they won't develop optimal tension. But of course, it isn't possible to truly eliminate one muscle group's contribution, only to lessen it.

Straight-leg hip extension unquestionably targets the hamstrings to a greater degree due to the fact that the hamstrings begin at normal length, but I've found that all bent-leg hip-extension exercises (think bridging derivatives here) also involve the hamstrings as a synergist. The difference with a bent-leg hamstring exercise is that the hamstrings are deliberately shortened to decrease their contribution and increase the contribution of the glute. With the knee bent, the length-tension relationship of the hamstrings is now poor and the glutes will be literally forced to do more work.

Hamstring cramps after bent-leg hamstring exercises clearly demonstrate that the person has poor glute function. In spite of the poor length-tension relationship, the hamstrings are still attempting to compensate for the weak glutes. The attempt to shorten an already deliberately shortened muscle causes that muscle to cramp.

The key to any of the hip-extension movements is to instruct the athlete to think "glutes first." Improvement of glute function must initially be a conscious effort.

As mentioned, there are still coaches who feel squatting is all the lower-body exercise an athlete needs. In reality, exercises such as squats and squat variations affect the glutes and hamstrings only as they relate to the knee and hip extension involved in achieving a neutral standing position. In squatting, the hip never moves into full extension. Quad-dominant athletes can become effective squatters with minimal glute involvement, particularly if allowed to squat to positions above parallel.

To properly work the glutes and hamstrings, the movement must be centered on the hip and not on the knee. To understand this concept, envision a front squat. The hip moves through an approximately 90-degree range of motion in concert with the knee movement.

Generally, there's one degree of hip movement for each degree of knee movement. The focus of the exercise is shared equally by the knee and hip extensors. In an exercise such as the single-leg straight-leg deadlift, the hip moves through a 90-degree range of motion, but the glutes are assisted by the hamstrings. A properly designed program must include both straight-leg hip-dominant exercises and bent-leg hip-dominant exercises to properly balance the lower-body muscles.

Beginners might be best off starting with the 8–10–12 bodyweight progression, meaning that only body weight is used for the first three weeks, but the number of repetitions increases each week, from 8 to 10 to 12 reps. External resistance may be used when appropriate.

What About Reverse Hypers?

It's amazing how quickly we can buy into an exercise without fully evaluating the movement, its orthopedic cost and its equipment space requirements. Louie Simmons and the Westside Barbell philosophy have turned many strength and conditioning coaches and personal trainers into reverse-hyper believers. I'll admit to jumping on the Louie bandwagon myself 20 years ago. For years, I had two reverse-hyper machines taking up lots of space and getting very little use.

In hindsight, I have a number of issues with reverse hypers:

I dislike buying equipment that only allows the performance of one exercise. At the end of the day, a reverse-hyper machine is just another single-station, single-joint machine that takes up a big chunk of space.

Reverse hypers work a non-functional pattern. The working leg should come from a hip- and knee-flexed position to a hip-extended position in locomotion. The pattern is hip flexion with accompanying knee flexion, followed by a multi-

joint extension of the hip and knee. In addition, we want the foot on the ground or at least pushing against something when we perform hip-extension exercises. In the case of the reverse hyper, the load is on the calf and Achilles.

Another huge problem is that as frequently demonstrated, reverse hypers actually feed synergistic dominance of the back extensors if not correctly taught and coached. In theory, the reverse hyper is performed by extending the hip with the glutes and hamstrings. This means lumbar extension shouldn't be the primary driver. In most cases, reverse hypers may actually feed dysfunction by allowing lumbar extension to substitute for hip extension. In most videos I've seen, the primary action is one of lumbar extension, with hip extension as a secondary action. If done correctly, we should see hip extension with a stable lumbar spine.

Lastly, reverse hypers aren't a particularly comfortable lift, particularly with heavy loads. The force on the stomach can be uncomfortable. This is conceptually similar to the barbell hip thrust, another popular internet exercise that's extremely uncomfortable.

The objective of powerlifting is to lift as much weight as possible. The reverse hyper is often sold as a primary assistance exercise for deadlifts. Deadlifts only require that the load moves from A to B. It doesn't matter which muscles do the work.

One reason I dislike conventional straight-bar deadlifts is that when done heavy, they're rarely done well. It's simply a fact of competitive powerlifting. As a former competitive powerlifter, I've watched thousands of deadlifts, and when the load gets heavy, the load gets shifted to the spinal erectors. This makes the lumbar-extension component of the reverse hyper attractive as an assistance exercise for powerlifting, but not for other athletes.

I've also never seen credible evidence that reverse hypers are effective in preventing or rehabilitating low-back pain. The concept of the reverse hyper is actually contrary to what many experts recommend for low-back pain. Our low-back protocols focus on keeping a stable lumbar spine while moving from the hip. This is generally more of a motor-control issue than a lumbar-erector strength issue.

Romanian Deadlift

I also admit to not being a fan of the double-leg versions of the straight-leg or Romanian deadlifts. Both lifts are difficult to teach, difficult to learn and have questionable applicability. Furniture moving comes to mind as a task that requires this lift.

I honestly believe that flexing from the hips with the spine stable—what physical therapists call a "waiter's bow" but is now the popular "hip hinge"—is one of the most difficult exercises to teach in strength and conditioning. Luckily, unlike squatting, very few athletes seem to miss modified straight-leg Romanian deadlifts if we take them out of the program.

As a result, we now use only single-leg versions of these exercises. Single-leg versions impact the back significantly less and impact the glutes and hamstrings both significantly and specifically more. The muscular systems of the deep longitudinal subsystem and lateral subsystem are trained far more effectively in the single-leg version. When we can obtain better muscular specificity and less lumbar load, that's clearly an improvement.

Old-school purists will wonder, "What, no RDLs?" But I'll always go back to the same point: If we can improve performance and have less chance of injury, I like the idea.

Single-Leg Straight-Leg Deadlift

The single-leg straight-leg deadlift is the staple of our posterior-chain program. It develops the entire posterior chain and enhances balance while decreasing both load and stress on the lower back.

This makes the exercise both extremely safe and extremely challenging. The tremendous proprioceptive work at the ankle is one of the less-obvious benefits of this deadlift. The deep longitudinal subsystem is engaged in this exercise, so the peroneals and tibialis anterior both must work hard to provide stability to the ankle, and consequently to the hip.

Not to be Captain Obvious, but single-leg hamstring work is more functional than double-leg hamstring work, and single-leg hamstring work that challenges balance and proprioception is the most beneficial. This is another exercise that can be used both as a part of the warm-up and as a loaded strength exercise.

Level 1—Reaching Single-Leg Straight-Leg Deadlift

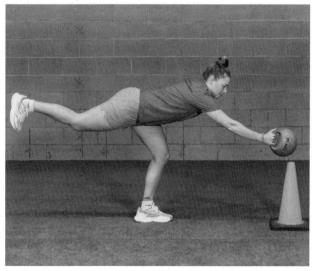

Figure 7.31—Reaching single-leg SLDL, a great way to teach the proper pattern.

To initially teach the single-leg straight-leg deadlift, we begin with a reaching version, particularly with children or adults who struggle with the pattern. The exercise is as simple as reaching for a cone while keeping the working leg semistraight—although straight is a misnomer, as the goal is 10–20% knee bend. Another advantage of the reaching version is that the thoracic extensors are engaged by the reach.

If a client struggles with balance, we move the cone outside the foot so the person has to reach across the body instead of straight ahead. Reaching across forces internal rotation of the pelvis against the femur, which creates greater glute recruitment (the same cross-body reach idea mentioned in the single-leg squat section).

The glute is both an extensor and an external rotator. Internal rotation stretches and activates the external rotator component of the glute max.

With beginners, we've done reaches for months until they master it. Getting a young athlete or an older client to move from the hip in a unilateral stance isn't easy.

It's also a big part of what we call "balance." I think the idea that one has bad balance is actually poor motor control of the deep longitudinal subsystem.

The inability to control the ankle, knee and hip is often viewed as a balance issue, but probably has little to do with the inner ear and lots to do with the knee and foot.

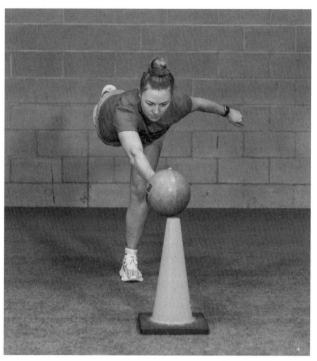

Figure 7.32—Regression 1, cross-body reach, much like the cross reach in a single-leg squat, the cross reach rotates the pelvis on a fixed femur.

Athletes generally begin with the reaching version and then progress to a single dumbbell or single kettlebell version.

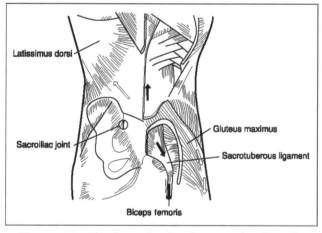

Figure 7.33—The thoracolumbar fascia is a key "transfer point" in hip-dominant unilateral exercises.

One-Dumbbell Single-Leg Straight-Leg Deadlift

One dumbbell or one kettlebell held opposite the working foot/leg further engages the anatomical subsystems. The key is to hold the load in the hand opposite the foot on the ground to force the opposite-side lat to work through the thoracolumbar fascia.

Think of the connection of glute and hamstrings through the thoracolumbar fascia, to the opposite-side lat. The goal is to have this entire system engaged to hold the load. We want to push this loading pattern until the athlete struggles with grip on the dumbbell or kettlebell. Our objective is to again "exhaust" the pure unilateral version before moving to two dumbbells or kettlebells.

Generally, the grip issue occurs at around 50% of body weight.

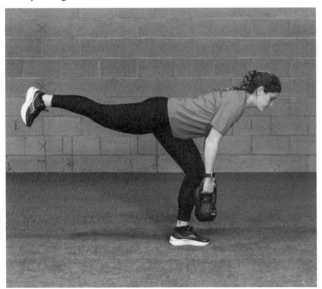

Figure 7.34—Two-dumbbell or two-kettlebell straight-leg deadlift.

The single-leg, two-arm straight-leg deadlift is the next step in the progression. The late Charles Poliquin frequently alluded to the idea of "varying the exercise without changing it." As Poliquin noted, the essence of the exercise remains the same, but the variation allows an increase in load.

The single-leg, two-arm straight-leg deadlift moves from a single dumbbell or kettlebell exercise to a two-dumbbell exercise and alters the loads at both the scapulothoracic joint and the thoracolumbar fascia. As mentioned, this allows greater loads than the single-arm version and will provide greater stress to all of the trunk extensors and scapula retractors, making the exercise an excellent progression from the single-dumbbell version.

From a functional standpoint, however, two dumbbells allow greater loads but may actually make the exercise less functional. I don't find this to be of great concern as the greater loads on the hip extensors offset the loss of the linkage from the glute max to the lat across the thoracolumbar fascia. The important point is that the person is able to progress with an increased load.

As before, we like to make this change when grip strength becomes an issue. Switching to two dumbbells or kettlebells allows the athlete to increase the load on the hip extensors, but the load may seem lighter. Progressing from a 70-pound dumbbell to a pair of 40s actually feels like a reduced load. Try it.

Slide Board Leg Curl

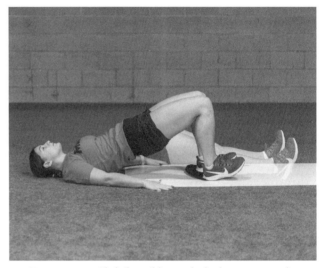

Figure 7.35—Slide board leg curl, the key is to use the hamstrings AND the glutes.

The slide board leg curl is an exercise stronger athletes can use as a level-one exercise, or it can be regressed to an eccentric-only exercise for beginners. The slide board leg curl has quickly become a favorite exercise even though it seems to violate the "no single-joint exercise" rule. In fact, the slide board leg curl isn't a single-joint exercise even though there's only one joint moving.

This leg curl works in a similar manner to hip-lift exercises. In any hip-lift exercise, the glute is the prime mover, while the hamstrings assist in hip extension. In the slide board leg curl, although only the knee joint is moving, the glute must act isometrically to keep the hip in extension. The hamstrings work to both eccentrically resist leg extension (a primary hamstring function) and concentrically produce knee flexion. This is a complex and functional exercise when performed correctly.

There's one major problem with the slide board leg curl. Previous authors who described this exercise with a stability ball made it a simultaneous hip flexion and knee flexion exercise where the hips are allowed to drop. This method takes what could be a great exercise and reduces it to an average exercise. The key to the slide board leg curl is that it forces the glutes and hamstrings to maintain hip extension while also using the hamstrings as both eccentric resistors of leg extension and then finally concentric knee flexors.

Eccentric-only version—Many trainees, particularly those who have glute control issues, won't be able to switch from the eccentric portion of the exercise to the concentric portion of the exercise while maintaining the glute contraction. In this case, the hips will drop and flex during the concentric portion of the exercise. If you see this, use eccentric-only reps to improve both strength and function.

You'll have your athlete start with the toes up and the heels on the board as in a double-leg bridge. Have him or her draw in the abdominals, and then place both hands on the glutes to feel the contraction. With both hands on the glutes and the stomach drawn in, ask for a five-second slide out combined with a hard exhale to go from the knee-flexed bridge position to a position with the legs straight. From that point, relax and return to the bridge position and repeat for three to five reps.

Concentric version—These are done as before but maintaining the glute contraction and leg curl back to the start position. It's critical that there's no bend at the hips.

Stability-Ball Leg Curl

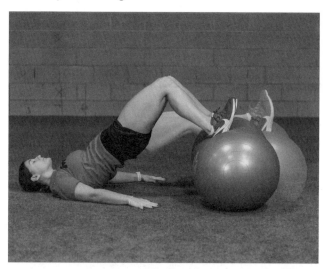

Figure 7.36—Peanut leg curl, a peanut-shaped ball is unstable in only one dimension.

The stability-ball leg curl is a more difficult progression because it requires using the glutes and spinal erectors to stabilize the torso and hamstrings to perform a closed-chain leg curl. This exercise develops torso stability while also strengthening the hamstrings. We've switched to "peanut balls" to make this exercise easier. A stability-ball leg curl with a peanut ball is easier than with a "normal" round ball and is easier than the slide board version.

Technique Points

• Heels are placed on the ball and the body is held with the hips off the ground.
• The ball is curled under the body using the heels, while the body is kept straight.

See page 113 of *New Functional Training for Sports* for further details.

CHAPTER 8
UPPER-BODY PULLING AND PRESSING

Upper-body pulling movements were covered in great detail in my first book, *Functional Training for Sports* and again in *Advances in Functional Training* and *New Functional Training for Sports*. The intention of this new book is to provide primarily new or updated information. In the case of upper-body pulling actions, not much has changed in recent years.

However, in most strength training programs, pulling movements such as chin-ups and rows still aren't given enough emphasis. I often see coaches and trainers who have their athletes and clients perform variations of lat pulldowns for the muscles of the upper back under the mistaken assumption that's all that's necessary. In addition, many programs still completely ignore rowing movements. This type of program design leads to the ever-present overdevelopment of the pressing muscles, which often lead to postural problems and eventually to shoulder injury.

A well-designed upper-body program should include a proportional ratio of sets of horizontal pulling (rowing) and vertical pulling (chin-up) to overhead pressing and supine pressing exercises. There should be a set of a pulling exercise for every set of a pushing exercise.

A poor ratio of pulling to pressing leads to overdevelopment of the pectorals and underdevelopment of the scapula retractors, which predisposes athletes to overuse shoulder injuries, especially rotator-cuff tendinitis. The incidence of rotator-cuff tendinitis among athletes who perform a great deal of bench press and bench press variations is extremely high. In truth, many powerlifters accept shoulder pain as a part of the sport in much the same way swimmers or tennis players do. But with a balanced program, very few athletes should experience anterior shoulder pain.

In my opinion, the anterior shoulder pain isn't due to the bench press itself, but rather to the lack of an appropriate ratio of pulling movements. The key is for athletes to possess an appropriate ratio of pulling to pushing strength. This is best estimated by comparing an athlete's maximum bench press to a calculated chin-up max. Athletes capable of bench pressing well over their body weight should also be capable of pulling well over their body weight, regardless of size.

For example:

> A 200-pound male athlete who can bench press 300 pounds should be able to perform 12 to 15 chin-ups and weighted chin-ups with 55 pounds for a minimum of five reps. Think of the chin-up as 255 x 5 (200 pounds of body weight plus 55 pounds of external load), roughly equivalent to a 300-pound bench press.

> A 300-pound male athlete who can bench press 400 pounds should be able to do five to eight chin-ups and five reps with a 25-pound plate (325 x 5).

Women generally perform better in the ratio of chin-up to bench press. We've found that female athletes capable of bench pressing their body weight can perform anywhere from 5 to 10 chin-ups and easily chin 25 pounds for five reps.

Vertical Pulling Movements

A properly designed strength program should include at least one chin-up variation each week, as well as a minimum of three sets of two different rowing movements per week.

The Charles Poliquin concept of varying the exercise without changing it applies particularly to the upper back. Either the specific type of vertical and horizontal pull should change every three weeks or the number of repetitions should change. In some cases, both should change.

Vertical pulling movements like chin-ups and chinning variations should be cycled in conjunction with horizontal pressing movements like the bench press. If you're assigning sets of three in the bench press, use sets of three in the vertical pulling movements too.

Our male athletes will rapidly gain upper-back strength with this type of program. It's not unusual for them to perform five chin-ups with a 45-pound plate attached to a dip belt.

Years ago, I called a belt manufacturer to inquire about dip belts in size 24 for small waists. When asked the purpose, I replied that these were for our female athletes to perform weighted chin-ups and pull-ups. Our female athletes frequently complained that the dip belts slid down due to the fact that the smallest belt was made for a 30-inch waist. The supplier stated that in all his years of belt manufacturing, he'd never been asked to make dip belts that size.

Just think of the name. We don't call them chin-up belts; we call them dip belts. The belts were designed to allow athletes to add weight for dips, not chin-ups. But it isn't unusual to walk into one of our facilities and see a female athlete or client performing sets of three chin-ups with anywhere from 5 to 45 pounds.

One of our female athletes, ice hockey World Champion and Olympian Alex Carpenter, has performed seven reps with a 45-pound plate hanging off a dip belt. She's also done 15 bodyweight chin-ups in testing.

Don't get caught in the trap of adding chin-ups to your program and then not training them as a strength exercise. Treat vertical pulling as a strength exercise and you'll see large increases in strength and subsequent decreases in shoulder pain.

Horizontal Pulling Movements

Horizontal pulling movements—these are rowing movements—are critical for two reasons:

The addition of rowing motions to the program will help prevent injury.

Rowing exercises are the true antagonistic movement to the bench press. Although chin-ups and their variations are important, rowing movements specifically target both the muscles and the movement patterns that directly oppose those trained on the bench press.

Despite their importance, rows are even more frequently omitted from strength programs than vertical pulling exercises. Rowing motions are an area of functional training that's undergoing great change. Recent advances in athletic training and physical therapy have shown the body is linked both anteriorly and posteriorly in diagonal patterns.

The posterior was discussed in great detail in chapter 7, but the information is also true in relation to rowing motions. Force is transmitted from the ground through the leg to the hip via the biceps femoris and the glute max. The force is then transferred across the sacroiliac joint into the opposite lat. The key in this system of cross-linkage lies not only in stabilizing the hip, but also in engaging the muscles used in the proper motor pattern.

For this reason, many rowing motions, with the exception of the inverted and rotational rows, are performed with one foot in contact with the ground. With a load in the hand opposite the foot on the ground, the person must now engage the biceps femoris and glute, the pelvic stabilizers (glute med, quadratus and adductors) and the hip rotators. The hip-rotator group and pelvic stabilizers are of particular importance because all force transferred from the ground must move through a stable hip to properly transfer to the upper body.

Until recently, the hip-rotator group has been mostly ignored. The hip rotators are the "rotator cuff" of the lower body, but they don't get the attention given to the shoulder rotator cuff muscles.

All force originating at the ground, whether a golf swing or a home run, must transfer through a strong, flexible and stable hip. Rowing exercises are covered in detail on pages 161–165 of *New Functional Training for Sports*. The exercises that follow are exercises that weren't in *Functional Training for Sports* or exercises we've updated.

Dumbbell Row

The dumbbell row is one of the simplest of rowing movements, yet it can be one of the most difficult to teach. This is a beginner level-one rowing exercise.

We've used a number of cues, props and progressions to teach dumbbell rows and can honestly say no single method or technique appears to be best. Although the exercise seems basic, like a simple case of "grab a dumbbell and pull," this couldn't be further from the truth.

A dumbbell row requires the person to position the hips and back properly prior to beginning. Getting in the start position and maintaining that position is the hardest part of the exercise.

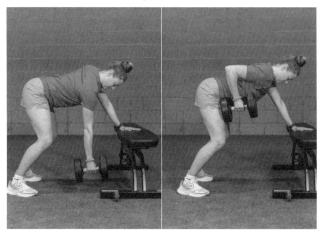

Figure 8.1—Dumbbell row (hand on the bench), dumbbell rows look simple but are amazingly hard to do and teach.

We begin with light weights so we can teach the proper hip position (a squat-type stance) and proper back position (slight arch) and then attempt to teach the movement while maintaining both those hip and back positions.

Athletes who can't touch their toes will have the most difficult time learning dumbbell rows. The ability to bend forward at the waist and then arch the back requires a degree of hamstring length. No amount of teaching will get an athlete with tight hamstrings into the proper position.

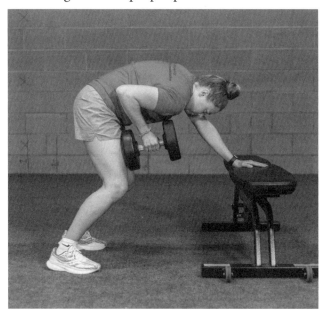

Figure 8.2—Dumbbell row, incorrect (back round, knees in), new trainees will often struggle to control the hips and core simultaneously.

Options

Two Feet on the Floor, Hand on the Bench—This is the version we try as step one. If an athlete can get into and maintain this position, there's no need for additional coaching or cueing. This is rare in our experience (particularly with adults and middle schoolers). We cue squat stance, wide knees and back arch. "Arched" usually gets us to flat, so this is a conscious "overcue." Often this deteriorates into a case of double valgus collapse and back rounding.

One Foot on the Floor, Same Side Hand and Knee on the Bench—For some trainees, this may solve the issue of pelvic position by allowing more arch. The bench also serves to anchor one leg, so a double-valgus collapse isn't possible.

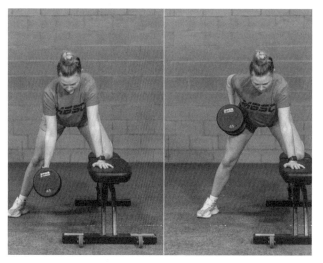

Figure 8.3—Dumbbell row, hand and knee on the bench— this variation can often help taller athletes.

Bench Straddle, Hand on Bench—I like this modification to reinforce the "squat stance." The feel of the bench against the leg reinforces the idea of wide knees. In all three versions, to perform the dumbbell row, your client will lean forward and place one hand on a bench to help stabilize the torso and take stress off the low back.

Teach the body position prior to pulling. The start position is a difficult position to hold. Have the athlete concentrate first on moving the scapula and then the elbow to bring the dumbbell back to the hip. I tell athletes that the back of the dumbbell should hit the hip bone at the iliac crest. Keep the weights light until you're confident in the setup.

Assign three sets of 5 to 10 reps, depending on the phase of the program.

Strength and Conditioning Coaching

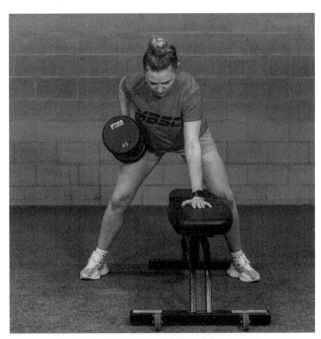

Figure 8.4—Dumbbell row, bench straddled—this variation will help athletes who collapse the knees.

Pressing Exercises: How Much Can You Bench?

That title is a little deceptive. The truth is, it doesn't matter how much people can bench. However, many athletes and coaches still believe the bench press is the measure of the success or failure of an athlete's off-season workouts.

I frequently see players making tremendous progress in pulling and in lower-body strength, but they're fixated on the bench press because, "Coach wants me up to 200 on the bench."

The logic that increases in bench press ability correlate with improvement of sport skill is flawed at best. The bench press is an indicator of one type of upper-body strength, a type that matters very little in most sports. However, this is a book on designing strength programs and if I don't give the bench press some attention, many coaches won't read or trust the book.

But, we use many exercises and movement patterns to develop strength. Don't judge a player's success or failure based on the bench press results.

So, why do coaches place such emphasis on the bench press?

> *The bench press is an easy exercise to do and test, much easier in both categories than an exercise like the hang clean. Bench press testing can be done rapidly and with very little teaching. However, increases in lower-body strength and power will have a far greater bearing on performance enhancement.*

> *Most athletes like to bench press and are willing to work at it. However, people generally like the bench press for all the wrong reasons. Athletes like the bench press because they see rapid improvements in muscles that are left over from our quadruped days. The pectoral muscles are somewhat left from when we walked on our hands. The reason we see such rapid change in the pecs from bench pressing is we literally "wake up" muscles that don't get used a lot. We go from atrophy to pecs in a few weeks. Coaches like this instant gratification. They like it when players look better.*

> *Most coaches have a limited knowledge of strength and conditioning and like most people, they assume we measure strength by how much can we bench. Start a conversation with any layman about workouts and the "how much" question will invariably come up.*

Is there a better way? Yes. Unfortunately, the truly beneficial exercises in strength training aren't as easy to learn. They take time, patience and coaching. Testing is difficult and potentially dangerous, but not impossible.

What's the solution?

> *Coaches should at least test performance-related factors like the 10-yard fly and the vertical jump, which are readily improved by good lower-body training. Remember, athletes will train for tests. Make the bench press the big test and you'll have athletes with big upper bodies and potentially no improvement in the ability to play their sports. One thing I can state clearly: Improvements in the 10-yard dash and vertical jump correlate strongly with improvements in performance.*

> *Coaches should start their teams on strength programs that emphasize*

lower-body and abdominal strength, and deemphasize the bench. Put your emphasis and your influence in the correct place.

In spite of the above, clients and coaches still want to know about upper-body strength—and about bench pressing in particular.

Horizontal pressing exercises like the bench press and its variations present a few interesting dilemmas. Many young athletes initially experience a rapid strength gain from a bench press program that's often done three times a week and features lots of "max" attempts. Due to the lack of relative use the muscle gets in normal life, training progress is rapid and some hypertrophy occurs quickly.

This creates a fundamental problem. The lifter associates the success with the frequency and intensity of workouts, not with the concept of awakening a long-dormant muscle. As a result, the trainee assumes a cause-and-effect relationship between training frequency and strength gain. This unfortunately leads to a long-term plateau and frustration on the part of the trainee when he or she is unable to continue to produce the rapid results.

As a former powerlifter, I tried every program imaginable to improve my bench press. It wasn't until I realized there was no relationship between training volume and strength gain that I began to make progress. In fact, the only relationship I found between volume and strength gain was negative. Most average trainees will make better gains on a reduced-volume program.

My search for strength initially led me to the "written by guys on drugs for other guys on drugs" programming. This is the standard muscle-magazine, internet junk. After realizing this type of training wasn't working for me, I began to read the writings of guys like Dr. Ken Leistner and later, Stuart McRobert. Both authors espoused abbreviated workouts along the line of the old high-intensity, one-set-to-failure school of thought. Both were also proponents of basic multi-joint free-weight exercises.

McRobert wrote extensively about strength and size development for what he referred to as "hardgainers" and for years published the *Hardgainer* magazine.

Reading the work of people like McRobert and Leistner and combining that with what we know about exercise physiology and human nature led me to the following concepts.

Keys to bench pressing success:

Bench press only once per week. Heresy, you say? Not really. If you analyze the workouts of most great bench pressers, most perform the actual lift only once a week. Beginners might do better with two bench press days, but think of this as technical motor learning.

Perform only two upper-body pressing workouts per week. More heresy? Again, talk to most strength athletes. You'll rarely see any who still perform three upper-body pressing workouts each week. Anthony Robbins says, "Success leaves clues." Look at the routines of successful athletes for your clues.

If your clients bench press less than 200 pounds, buy a set of 1.25-pound Olympic plates. As they progress, the 5-pound jumps necessitated by 2.5-pound plates will be too large. If they bench over 200 pounds, you can get away with five-pound jumps, but 2.5s will still be better.

Work hard on the assistance exercises. Very often, plateaus in the bench press can be broken by increasing strength in the incline or close-grip bench press.

The reason athletes usually fail to improve their bench press after the first year is that they don't follow those rules. It's difficult to get people to stop doing something that's been successful, but in strength training, less is clearly more as trainees become more experienced.

The following will help you choose appropriate weights for your athletes or clients on the bench press assistance exercises. It's been my experience that most athletes don't push themselves in assistance exercises like they do in the bench press. So, we developed these charts so we could accurately predict what our athletes should be capable of in major dumbbell exercises.

If I have an athlete who can bench press 275 pounds, I expect that same athlete will be able to perform dumbbell bench presses with 85-pound dumbbells for 10 reps. Some readers might find this unusual, but if you look at the ratios, it's feasible.

1 RM 10 RM DB Bench 10RM
Bench Press 275 215 85

To determine dumbbell loads, we take 50 percent of the corresponding rep max load. In the above case, this would be 107.5 pounds. We then work off the assumption that an experienced athlete can handle 80 percent of a comparable barbell load with dumbbells, so we multiply 107.5 x .8 and get 86.

We'll generally only perform one horizontal pressing exercise per day. Most often, some type of pure horizontal pressing exercise will be done on the first day, like a bench press or a dumbbell bench press. On the second day, we'll use an incline or close-grip variation.

We see people who become extremely proficient at one exercise, but don't have proportional multi-angle strength. One of our upper-body goals is to have this balance between presses and between pressing and pulling. I don't want someone who's great at the bench press but can't incline press with a bar or handle heavy dumbbells.

I've read nearly everything there is to read in the field of strength and conditioning, and everyone from Doug Hepburn to Fred Hatfield made similar recommendations. The key to bench press success isn't in doing more exercises. The key is well-thought-out progressions and volume control. Stuart McRobert likes to say,

"If you are not getting stronger, your strength program isn't working."

Simple but powerful logic.

McRobert and many authors like him tell us that very few trainees who are serious aren't just doing enough—they're doing too much. Oddly, some of the strongest guys in every gym seem to be the laziest. They come in, do a few sets and leave. But they understand how to get strong. Getting stronger is about progression. It has nothing to do with getting bigger or getting a pump.

Why We've Moved Away From Bars

No, this isn't a story about my personal struggles. It's an explanation of why we've chosen dumbbells and individual pulley handles over straight bars.

For a long time, the barbell ruled. Straight-bar bench, back and front squats, and straight-bar deadlifts were the norm. Things like dumbbell bench press, dumbbell incline press and goblet squats were either ignored or viewed as accessory or auxiliary lifts.

However, over the last two decades, we moved away from fixed bars in almost every lift we do. The two exceptions are the hang clean and the bench press. Our "squat" racks have become bench press stations and pull-up bars, and we rarely see a bar in the rack at chest height.

What Happened?

Over the years, we realized that for a bunch of reasons, the straight bar isn't the best choice. Our process is simply to move away from the "this is the way it was always done" mentality and progress to thinking in a more logical fashion.

The book *Think Like a Freak* contains this quote:

"The conventional wisdom is often wrong and a blithe acceptance of it can lead to sloppy, wasteful or even dangerous outcomes."

Stop and think about that for a minute. For us in the strength field, it means changing some of our thoughts about the lifts.

Deadlifts

We exclusively trap bar deadlift, although some people like the term "hex bar deadlift." I've talked about this numerous times, but for us the trap bar made the straight bar obsolete as it applies to the deadlift. The ability to be "inside" the bar makes the lift far easier to teach and perform. It seems like only powerlifting purists continue to hang on to the straight-bar deadlift.

Pressing

The bench press is one exercise we kept, primarily out of convention. Athletes love the bench press, and I honestly think it would be bad for business if we eliminated it from our athlete programs. However, our adult clients never press a straight bar on any exercise (including the bench press) unless they specifically ask. We never do a straight-bar bench press, incline or overhead in any of our adult programming. In our athlete program, the only straight-bar press is the bench press.

The exception? Beginners. I still prefer bars to dumbbells for beginners. It's less neurologically complex to control a bar than attempt to control two dumbbells.

There are two major benefits to dumbbells over barbells in pressing.

Having to independently balance and control two dumbbells is better, plain and simple. The ability to compensate is taken away or drastically reduced.

Dumbbells are shoulder-friendly. The shoulder joint seems to self-select a path that's most comfortable when using dumbbells. This isn't as achievable with a straight bar. Although we may be able to play with shoulder angles when using a bar, we lose the ability to rotate the dumbbells in the transverse plane.

Squatting

This is easy because we eliminated back squats years ago. Beginners start with press-out squats or goblet squats. There are a number of reasons this is an improvement.

Both press-out squats and goblet squats have a self-limiting effect. They're hard to do wrong and in fact they *make* people do things right.

Getting a bar into the front or back squat position may be a mobility challenge, particularly for an adult client.

Pulling

We still do chin-ups and parallel-grip chin-ups with athletes from a "normal" chin-up bar. However, with the advent of functional trainers and suspension trainers, we've moved to independent hand grips for pulldowns and rows. In the case of pulldowns on a functional trainer or suspension rows, the shoulder can easily move from internal rotation to external rotation.

I often describe the shoulder as a spiral diagonal joint. The shoulder seems to function better when not prevented from moving through rotation.

To sum up, straight bars go a long way toward determining bar paths. I'm not sure that's a good thing for human joints, particularly shoulder joints.

Alternating Dumbbell Bench Press and Alternating Dumbbell Incline Press

From a functional training standpoint, there are two somewhat unconventional exercises I want to cover because alternating and incline dumbbell bench presses are significant improvements over the conventional variations due to the unilateral support and diagonal core load they provide.

In both movements, the dumbbells are supported at the top and alternated from the top. By performing these exercises in this manner, we develop considerable shoulder stability. The arm that's not pressing is working isometrically to maintain position while the working arm performs the pressing action.

In addition, the core is forced to create great diagonal stability to counter the force created by lowering one dumbbell at a time, whereas in symmetrical lifting, there's very little core loading. These two exercises take a routine upper-body pressing action and add two important dimensions.

New Functional Training for Sports covers additional horizontal pressing exercises. Again, the intent of the book you're reading is to add to the concepts in *New Functional Training for Sports*, not repeat information, so I won't repeat the material.

The key in horizontal pressing exercises isn't to focus solely on how much an athlete can bench press, but rather to develop well-rounded upper-body strength in the bench press, incline press and dumbbell variations.

As strength and conditioning coaches, we need to work to decrease the fascination with performing and evaluating one lift as if it's the only indicator of upper-body strength. You'll be amazed how few athletes can do 25 strict pushups. Don't lose sight of the ability to handle body weight.

CHAPTER 9
CHOOSING A SYSTEM OF TRAINING

Most coaches don't choose a system of training; their system seems to choose them. Coaches tend to either follow the crowd, follow their own training preferences or follow their own personal strength and conditioning experience. I advocate that you do none of that. Instead, I'll discuss the evolution of training systems and provide some insights into the pros and cons of each. I want you to take pieces where applicable to form a workable system for your clients and athletes.

Set and Rep Schemes

For beginners, there's too much emphasis on finding the perfect system of sets and reps. In reality, programming is not nearly as important as execution. In my experience, many high school and college coaches use advanced set-and-rep schemes and then implement these schemes with poor attention to technique. This is a huge mistake. KISS: Keep It Simple Stupid.

We should be strength and conditioning coaches, not computer geeks or periodization junkies. I use Excel spreadsheets with my more advanced athletes, but the ongoing trend of advanced programming done poorly is disturbing. You're only as good as the technical proficiency of your athletes.

Is Periodization Strength and Conditioning's Biggest Time Waster?

In *The Little Black Book of Training Wisdom*, Dr. Dan Cleather defines periodization as simply, "the planning and organization of training." Yet periodization has become so much more than that for some coaches.

I must confess I struggle to understand the concepts of periodization. Linear? Undulating? Concurrent? Conjugate?

Much of the periodization confusion comes from fascination of the Westside Barbell philosophy by many in our field. Westside advocates conjugate

periodization, a term many, including me, struggle to understand.

But the single differentiating factor for me is that training athletes isn't like training powerlifters. This is a basic problem. Powerlifters are athletes, but athletes aren't powerlifters. Trying to integrate the training concepts used by elite powerlifters into the training of athletes is difficult and potentially counterproductive.

Years ago I asked physical therapist Bill Hartmann to help clear up the terms for me. Bill stated:

"Concurrent is training multiple qualities simultaneously.

"Conjugated = linked.

"Conjugate is a variant of concurrent programming that still trains multiple qualities, but with an emphasis on one (greater portion of total training volume) while maintaining the others with limited volume in each training block. The point I think a lot of folks miss is that each preceding training block of emphasis is designed to enhance the following, which makes it conjugated…linked.

"For example, if a high-level athlete requires greater power output, a block emphasizing increased volume of maximal strength/maintaining power, followed by a reduction in volume of maximal strength work, and an increased emphasis/volume of power should raise power to a higher level than if both are worked equally in consecutive training blocks."

As I thought about these definitions, I realized why I was confused. In a sports training setting, we're always concurrent or conjugate. We constantly, out of necessity, train multiple quantities, but unlike powerlifters, we're seeking more than strength. A powerlifter's end goal is always strength.

113

Powerlifters may add dynamic days to attempt to develop explosiveness, but at the end of the day, the goal is simply to lift more weight.

When I began to understand the concepts better, I realized that training athletes is always concurrent and sometimes conjugate. The reason I failed to understand the concepts was because I'd been doing conjugate or concurrent periodization for 20 years. I just didn't know it.

We train for power at least three different ways. Our Olympic lifts and weighted jumps use heavy external loads to train for power, while plyometrics use primarily body weight. Medicine balls feature relatively light external loads in comparison to the significant loads used in jumps and Olympic lifting.

While I'm training an athlete for power, I'm concurrently training the athlete for strength. At certain times (notably pre-season), we might decrease the strength and power emphasis (are we now conjugate?) and have a greater energy system emphasis. Another concurrent thread?

On an interesting note, I listened to Al Vermeil on the Strengthcoach podcast, and Al simply said,

*"Keep a thread of everything
in your program."*

As soon as he said it, I stopped my car and wrote it in my notebook. Take your pick, concurrent or conjugate. I'm still not sure. The bottom line in sports training is that we can never train just for strength or just for power or just for speed. We need to train concurrently for all of the above in the off-season and keep at least a thread of all of it in the program year-round.

People make things so complicated that I needed help from Bill Hartmann to clarify things, and then a reminder from Coach Vermeil to "keep it simple."

Autoregulation?

Recently, I read a quote about "autoregulating loads based on readiness." More confusion? Author Eric Helms describes autoregulation this way:

"Autoregulation, simply put, is just a struc-tured approach for embedding a respect for individual variation within a program."

Autoregulation in this context sounds like a long euphemism for "well-coached strength training."

Questions like, "How do you feel?" come to mind. However, Helms was quick to point out that in his opinion, autoregulation isn't "training by feel."

If it's not training by feel, we again seem to end up in a bit of a semantics argument. If an idea like autoregulation doesn't come down to basing training on how an individual feels that day, I'm more confused than ever. Either way, we still seem to be fascinated with big words when it comes to program design.

Then another term came across my desktop. A Strengthcoach.com member asked for info on "daily undulating periodization." My question was once again, "What's that?" I needed to look up that one. Then I realized daily undulating periodization had formerly been called undulating periodization and might be more aptly named "weekly undulating periodization" because rep ranges are alternated during the week.

Alwyn Cosgrove referred to this simply as undulating periodization in a Strengthcoach.com article a few years ago. However, when I think of undulating periodization, I think of the Charles Poliquin idea of alternating phases of accumulation (increased volume) and intensification (increased load).

Really, we have so many conflicting or overlapping terms and ideas, I struggle to even find the definitions, much less understand what the author means by the term. In each case, the proponents seem to think their idea is "the one."

What Works?

A coach's need to create variation seems to be an exercise in self-stimulation. I tell our coaches we should be writing programs to develop our athletes and not to stimulate ourselves. As coaches, we want to prove our worth so we study and study, looking for the Holy Grail of programming. But there may not *be* a Holy Grail of programming.

Chris Doyle used to say that the best program may be the one we aren't on. The best program might be the next one, provided it's not the same as the last one.

What works, in my experience, is a combination of progressive resistance exercise and a progression and regression system.

In the early 1980s, the late Charles Poliquin wrote the best article I've read on periodization—it was called "Variety in Strength Training." Poliquin advocated undulating periodization versus the traditional Mike Stone/John Garhammer linear periodization model.

The undulation in the Poliquin plan isn't weekly, but rather every three weeks. Loads are increased slightly each week (we tend to use 2.5%), and rep ranges or contraction emphasis are changed every three weeks. Undulating periodization is simply alternating what Poliquin called "periods of accumulation" (more volume and/or time under load) versus "periods of intensification" (higher loads and lower reps).

The key in the Poliquin system is a wave-like approach, literally an undulation that creates gradual upward progress. This became my definition of undulating periodization, a wave-like variation of the earlier Stone/Garhammer step-type models of linear periodization.

When it comes to training, change is good; progressive resistance is good and small plates are good. For well over 30 years, our athletes have developed incredible strength and power with the Poliquin undulating model in combination with the Stuart McRobert concept of small plates and small increases.

Our facilities have lots of 1.25- and 2.5-pound plates, and we use them. Depending on the person, the goal is something as simple as doing one more rep at the same load or adding 2.5 pounds (1.25 on each side) for the same number of reps.

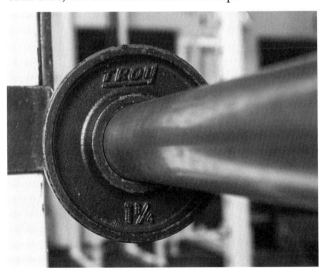

Figure 9.1—1.25-pound plate—if you want to make continual progress, purchase some 1.25s.

Trust me, the real periodization secret is, there is no secret. Spend more time coaching and prescribing precise loads and less time wondering which magic periodization formula works best.

Keep it simple stupid. I tell people MISS and KISS: Make it simple; Keep it simple.

The Simplest Method: Progressive Resistance Exercise (PRE)

The simplest method of progression for beginners is simply to add weight to the bar or add reps with the same weight. The only stipulation is that the athlete performs the exercises with perfect technique. This is basic progressive resistance exercise (PRE).

More experienced lifters add 2.5 pounds per week to the heaviest set. This is a simple system advocated by the old HARDgainer crowd.

Less-experienced lifters perform the same weight for one more rep each week.

> Stuart McRobert was the publisher of HARDgainer in the 1980s and he wrote two excellent books, *Brawn* and *Beyond Brawn*. McRobert's philosophy was wonderful in its simultaneously innovative yet simple approach. I'm a huge McRobert fan, and early in my career I read everything he wrote.

Many so-called big-time strength coaches reject this type of programming as too simple, but this simple PRE program forms the basis of almost all of our training from kids to pros. Periodization is fairly minimal, and we employ PRE almost exclusively. The advantages of a simple progressive exercise program are evident:

The system works extremely well with beginners and may be all they'll ever need.

PRE can be combined with other methods, like Poliquin's undulating periodization, for a simple periodized program.

Generally, we perform one or two work sets per exercise after the warm-up sets.

The sequence is as follows—a warm-up set first, heavy set second, heavy set plus or minus 5 to 10 pounds third. With the third set, the coach decides whether the athlete goes up, down or stays at the same weight. Obviously, stronger athletes may need more warm-up sets, but not more work sets.

Picking Set Three

One thing that comes up a lot in our coaches' meetings is the "how" of choosing weights for athletes. It's sort of like the story of *Goldilocks and the Three Bears*. We don't want the weight to be too heavy or too light. We want it to be just right.

In the perfect heavy set, the last rep looks like, well, the last rep. In a perfect world, you know the athlete probably couldn't get one more rep. With a perfectly selected load, there's no need for a spotter and also no need to think, "We could have gone with five more pounds."

We talk about the process of picking what weight to do next as the intersection of the science of strength training and the art of coaching. To envision what I mean, imagine you just watched an athlete complete the first work set of a planned three-set workout, remembering that workouts for us are usually a warm-up set followed by two work sets.

After watching the set, you have three choices:

You can have the athlete increase the weight— often by 2.5 pounds using 1.25-pound plates, but rarely by more than 5 pounds if you're good at selecting the first work set.

You can have the athlete use the same weight on the next set.

You can decrease the weight. If we decrease, I'll always go down by at least 5 pounds and will rarely use the 1.25-pound plates for a decrease.

Hit it right, and you're a genius. Hit it wrong, and the athlete fails.

When making the decision to go up, down or repeat, keep the same vision in mind: *The last rep should look like the last rep.*

This is where experience as a lifter comes in and for this reason, I want my coaches to train themselves. Experienced lifters instinctively know what that next set should be. They can tell whether to go up, down or repeat.

Reminder, male athletes' egos are much more developed than their muscles. They'll always say, "I can do more." You have to select the load not based on their desire or ego, but on your experience. Female athletes can often do the opposite and underestimate their ability.

In the cases of young men, the answer will often be to repeat the same weight or go down in weight. For young women, the answer might be a 2.5-pound increase using 1.25-pound plates.

The most important lesson is that slow and steady wins the race. Any time you think you're being too conservative, remind yourself that 5 pounds per week for 10 weeks is 50 pounds. Don't be greedy.

On the flip side, 5 pounds is 10 percent of 50 pounds. Going up by 5 pounds for a weaker athlete is a huge jump. Five is to 50 as 30 is to 300. Think about that when you tell a younger or weaker athlete to go up 10 pounds. Remind yourself it's not the amount but the percentage.

Choosing weights and creating a challenging environment for athletes may be one of the most important coaching skills a young coach can learn. Coaches need to develop a thought process that allows them to make the right decision to positively impact the long-term success of each athlete.

By following a simple program of progressive resistance exercise, you could theoretically improve 260 pounds per year. While no athlete will make five-pound weekly increases for an entire year, most athletes would be happy with much smaller gains than 260 pounds in any lift.

In theory, an athlete who's able to hang clean an empty 45-pound bar for five reps would be cleaning 95 pounds for five reps by week 10. By week 20, this means cleaning 145 for five reps. Some of our female athletes have become incredibly strong by using this simple system.

5–6–7–8–9 for Kids

One thing I love about training a broad spectrum of clients and athletes is that I'm always learning. Just when I think I have all the answers, there are more questions. It's always been perplexing to figure out how to move kids up in weight while maintaining good technique and avoiding plateaus. It's not as simple as the idea of the progressive resistance exercise previously discussed.

In a collegiate environment, we just throw five more pounds on the bar and go for it. It's pretty simple. Five pounds a week can really add up for a college athlete.

But what do you do with a kid who's bench pressing 45 pounds for five reps? Adding five pounds at this point increases the load by about 12% and could cause a host of problems.

We've used the 1.25-pound Olympic plates with some success. However, that idea is effective but not foolproof. In training middle school athletes, we're still experiencing plateaus even when using 1.25-pound plates. And we run into issues with dumbbells and kettlebells where our smallest possible jump is generally 2.5 pounds for dumbbells or two kilograms per hand for kettlebells.

So, we found another solution, which I know sounds simple: Instead of increasing weight, we increase reps. Once one of the kids begins to hit a bit of a wall, we switch from increasing weight to increasing reps.

A three-week goblet squat phase might be 80 x 5, 80 x 6, 80 x 7. I've taken to using five-week phases with my kids' group—just going 5–6–7–8–9,

then moving up to the next dumbbell or plate and repeating the sequence.

Try it. I think you'll like it.

I've had kids progress in the bench press from 100 x 5 to 100 x 9 with no plateaus, and I have a 14-year-old young woman goblet squatting 80 x 9.

These kinds of revelations, gained through well-founded experimentation, are perhaps why one of my favorite quotes is, "It's what you learn after you know it all that counts."

Training Methods

American engineer and business theorist Harrington Emerson stated:

"As to methods there may be a million and then some, but principles are few. The man who grasps principles can successfully select his own methods. The man who tries methods, ignoring principles, is sure to have trouble."

Let's take a look at some of the methods used in strength and conditioning.

Four-Phase Undulating Periodization Model (Poliquin Model)

	PHASE 1	INTENSITY	VOLUME	PHASE 2	INTENSITY	VOLUME
REPS	3 x 8	60–77%	24	4–6 x 3	90–97%	12–18
TEMPO	Varied: Eccentric / Pause / Concentric Ex. 3/1/1					

	PHASE 3	INTENSITY	VOLUME	PHASE 4	INTENSITY	VOLUME
REPS	3–5 x 5	80–87%	15–25	4–6 x 3	90–97%	12–18
TEMPO	Varied: Eccentric / Pause / Concentric Ex. 3/1/1					

As I mentioned, Poliquin's work in the 1990s caused me to rewrite all of my workouts. After contemplating the concept of paired exercises, the conclusion was obvious: Paired exercise sequences make better use of time. In the Poliquin method, practicality becomes an issue due to equipment availability. Care must be taken to make sure athletes are pairing the correct exercises—more on that later.

The Westside System

The favored system of the masses still seems to be a Louie Simmons Westside Barbell approach centered around powerlifting-style training. Although Mr. Simmons made some wonderful contributions to the field, for a variety of reasons, I can't advocate most of the methods.

The reasons are simple:

Although he presented his training as evidence- and results-based, it may actually be neither. There's no independent research I've seen that validates the training concepts advocated by Westside.

In fact, most of the evidence the Westside system points to is tainted by the use of performance-enhancing drugs.

The Westside system is designed to produce powerlifters, not athletes. Powerlifting is a sport consisting of three lifts: the squat, bench press and deadlift. The essence of the Westside system revolves around improving these three lifts. The not-so-logical conclusion is that improvement in the three powerlifts leads to improved sports performance.

Although in a simplistic sense, the improvement of force production will produce some changes, our knowledge of functional anatomy leads us to conclude that training for sports must be more specific and improve strength quantities unique to the single-leg nature of most sports.

On the other hand, Simmons, like Stone and Poliquin, must be recognized for pushing the envelope and redefining the sport of powerlifting. His ideas about speed of movement and variable resistance were the first advances in training for strength in a long time.

My objection to the variable-resistance methods he proposed doesn't lie in my belief that the methods don't work, but in practical concerns. Simmons' two most significant contributions are in the use of bands and chains for variable resistance.

Chains are a great concept, but they're expensive and somewhat time-consuming to use. In simple terms, heavy chains are attached to the bar, so as the bar is lowered, the chain gathers on the floor—the weight is reduced by the amount of chain accumulating on the floor. As the bar is raised, the weight increases as the chain comes off the floor. This is an ingenious concept of applying variable resistance to a free weight environment, where the load more closely matches the strength curve and allows the lifter to accelerate the bar. However, this can be impractical to set up and somewhat expensive for groups.

Another Simmons innovation is the use of heavy elastic bands to provide resistance similar to the chain idea. Bands are anchored to the power rack and then placed around the ends of the bar. As the load is lowered, the band decreases in elastic energy and the load becomes lighter. As the lifter raises the bar, the load again increases due to the tension placed on the band. This is again free weight used in a variable-resistance environment.

It's also a stroke of genius, but it requires a coach to purchase bands, and more importantly, to monitor the condition of the bands. A broken band in this situation could be disastrous.

Simmons' methods are brilliant, but besides being empirical in nature, they can be costly, time-consuming and, in the case of bands, potentially dangerous. This doesn't discount his brilliance, but it does make these methods somewhat questionable from a practical standpoint.

The idea of using a single sport like powerlifting or Olympic lifting to train for another sport is a well-intentioned idea, but probably not a sound concept. Coaches can take some concepts from the Westside Barbell school of thought to help an athlete improve in the bench press, and may utilize concepts from the training of Olympic lifters to help an athlete improve in the hang clean, but all of these concepts must eventually meet to help the athlete better produce and reduce force on one leg.

A program of Olympic weight-lifting or powerlifting won't provide the proper musculoskeletal stresses necessary to truly improve sport performance.

The critics will say this isn't true, but I'd say it's half true.

To most efficiently and effectively improve sport performance, athletes need to work in single-leg environments unlike those contested in sports like Olympic lifting or powerlifting. Lifts like the squat, bench press and hang clean might be part of the solution, but must be complemented with specific exercises to develop the single-leg extension patterns of the hip and knee.

CrossFit and Other High-Intensity Functional Systems: Why CrossFit May Not Be Good for Your Clients

Let's face it, CrossFit is a controversial topic in the world of strength and conditioning. CrossFit gyms are cheap and easy to open, with only a weekend certification and a few thousand dollars worth of equipment. This appeals to many people in the fitness business. You can be part of what WAS a rapidly growing trend, and you can do it without great expense. I'm not a CrossFit fan, but I will try to keep my personal opinions to myself and deal with what's generally agreed upon as safe in strength and conditioning.

I knew very little about CrossFit until 2005 when I was contacted by representatives of SOMA, the Special Operations Medical Association. CrossFit was their concern, not mine. I was asked to come to the SOMA meeting in Tampa, Florida, to discuss training special operations soldiers. At a panel discussion, I offered answers to questions asked about CrossFit and the controversy began.

What follows isn't from the SOMA meeting, but are my thoughts since then.

Major Question 1—Is planned randomization a valid concept? CrossFit is based on the idea that the workouts are planned, but are deliberately random. I think the term "planned randomization" is an oxymoron. Workouts are either planned or random.

I strongly believe that workouts should be planned and that a specific progression should be followed to prevent injury. The Workout of the Day (WOD) idea is fundamentally flawed.

Major Question 2—Is training to failure safe? CrossFit is, at its base, a competitive or self-competitive program in which it becomes necessary to train to failure.

There are two layers of problems here. The first is the simple question of whether training to failure is beneficial to the trainee. Some strength and conditioning experts believe training to failure is beneficial; others caution against it. Now, I like training to failure, but this brings up the larger question of what constitutes "failure."

The late Charles Poliquin (another non-CrossFit fan) popularized the previously mentioned term "technical failure," and this is the definition we adhere to. Technical failure occurs not when the person is no longer capable of doing the exercise, but when the person is unable to perform the exercise with proper technique. In training beyond technical failure, the stress shifts to tissues that weren't and probably shouldn't be the target of the exercise.

The third layer of questioning training to failure relates to what movements lend themselves to the style. In the area of "generally agreed as safe," high-velocity movements like Olympic lifts and jumps aren't done to failure and never should be taken beyond technical failure.

Is it one bad rep or multiple bad reps? How many bad reps are too many?

Major Question 3—Is an overuse injury (generally an injury caused by repeated exposure to light loads) different from an overstress injury (an injury caused by exposure to heavy loads)? Both are injuries. The first is overuse; the second is trauma. In my mind, injuries are injuries…period.

Major Question 4—Should adults be Olympic lifters? This is a big one. I don't think Olympic lifts are good for adults. Most adults can't get their arms safely over their head once, much less 50 times under load.

The other question that begs to be asked is, should anyone do high-rep Olympic lifts? The best Olympic lifters in the world say no.

With all that said, believe it or not, my biggest problem is actually less with the workouts than it is with the false bravado and character assassination of dissenters. The CrossFit community can be pretty venomous when their concepts are questioned.

It's also filled with people who think injury is a normal part of the training process. I've spoken up against endurance athletes who willingly hurt themselves and to me, there's no difference between that and the CrossFit controversy.

I know this will generate more controversy, but CrossFit might be the biggest controversy in strength and conditioning since HIT training.

Bodybuilding Method

In spite of advances made in the field of strength and conditioning, social media has sparked an increase in interest in the bodybuilding method. Generally, coaches using a bodybuilding method to train their athletes were ex-bodybuilders simply using what they learned in their own training. This is an extremely inefficient method for athletes, since bodybuilding, like powerlifting and Olympic lifting, is a sport more than an actual training system.

"Bodybuilding" is characterized by high-volume workouts generally broken into body parts. It has very little athletic application and is often time-consuming due to a multi-angular approach.

The idea of bodybuilding frequently results in misplaced emphasis, as the aim of a competitive bodybuilder is improved appearance, not improved performance. Bodybuilding can also be extremely counterproductive for those looking to lose weight because the high-volume workouts might potentially result in muscle hypertrophy. However, bodybuilding may be helpful to athletes who need to gain additional mass.

As previously mentioned, social media has reignited interest in bodypart training, particularly with young males. In high school, strength and conditioning coaches will often have to "deprogram" young males who believe that bodypart training will lead to the perfect physique.

Olympic Lifting

Much like the Westside system, some coaches espoused or adopted a philosophy based on the sport of Olympic weightlifting. This is another example of athletes being trained in one sport to hopefully improve their ability in a different sport. This is conceptually no different than the Westside approach.

Olympic lifting is a sport. Attempting to train other athletes like Olympic weightlifters is often like putting a square peg in a round hole. What makes a good Olympic weightlifter from the standpoint of a lever system may not make a great lineman or power forward.

High Intensity Training

I include information about high intensity training because at other points in the book, I've referred to it by name. High intensity training or HIT, as it's come to be called, is the brainchild of Nautilus inventor Arthur Jones and is an extremely interesting phenomenon in the world of strength and conditioning.

Although the system appears to have a limited basis in exercise physiology, high intensity training has an extremely long history and a loyal and dedicated following.

There are a few varieties of high intensity programming. Proponents ranged from professional strength and conditioning coaches who believed strongly in the original Nautilus philosophy of one set to momentary muscular failure done on a circuit of 12 to 15 machines, to people like the late Ken Leistner and Stuart McRobert, who advocate a similar philosophy based on basic free weight movements. All of the proponents of HIT share a belief that less is more, and I probably have more in common with these folks and have been more heavily influenced by them than I'd like to admit.

The proponents of HIT believe in very hard, very brief work. The problem with this type of system is the zeal borders on fanaticism. HIT is a small but interesting splinter group in the world of strength and conditioning that should be investigated before it's totally discounted. There's clearly a mental benefit to asking athletes to work to complete failure. I believe the HIT system will work well in team sports settings where intrinsic motivation is an issue.

My major point of disagreement with the proponents of HIT lies in their stance on power development. In classic HIT, no power work is performed. Proponents believe moving a load with speed is inherently dangerous. As a result, neither plyometrics nor Olympic lifts were used in the original HIT workouts. My feeling is that the work of exercise physiologists in the area of the stretch-shortening cycle and the force-velocity curve made this stance difficult to defend.

Proponents of HIT believe we should lift for strength and then simply practice sport skills, and that there's no neurological middle ground. Some proponents of HIT, particularly in the collegiate world, are beginning to use plyometrics to develop the stretch-shortening cycle, although many of the early proponents saw no need for stretch-shortening exercises.

My Conclusion

No single system provides all the answers. A sound training program will take strength development ideas from powerlifting, power development ideas from Olympic lifting, speed improvement ideas from track and injury prevention concepts from physical therapy. The integration of these disciplines may lead to the ultimate program.

The most important element in program design is to choose a system you understand and choose exercises you're comfortable teaching.

CHAPTER 10
CREATING EFFICIENT AND EFFECTIVE WORKOUTS

Having training knowledge is one thing. Being able to take that knowledge and use it to design a program is another thing entirely. The key to being able to design great training programs lies in the ability to filter information.

You can't make a big program change every time a new idea comes across your desk—you need to look at new information and filter out the hype.

One Big Change

Over my entire career, I've been a "day one is lower-body day" coach. The reasoning behind this traces back to the days when attendance at off-season programs was voluntary. My feeling was that the first day you showed up would be a lower-body day because if athletes only made three of the recommended four days, they'd get two lower-body days, and if they only came once, they'd get one good lower-body day.

From a psychological perspective, this also meant most athletes would get a minimum of two days. My early clients were mostly American football players, and they rarely missed a bench press day, which was on day two.

It was a mind game, like "You can't have dessert until you clean your plate." You can't bench if you don't squat first. This was, of course, back when we were squatting like everyone else.

The point is, I carried my old ideas much longer than I should have and wore my "lower-body first" idea as a badge of honor.

Arizona Cardinals' Reconditioning Coach Buddy Morris finally convinced me to change. I heard Buddy on a podcast say:

"I have no idea what my players did or where they were over the weekend. I could have guys flying back from Vegas or Miami late Sunday or even Monday morning. I couldn't have my most important day be Monday."

As a result, this edition of this book will be the first edition where I flip the four-day template to start the week with an upper-body day.

I firmly believe the more time you can spend with your athletes, the better the results will be. For this reason, I'm a proponent of four-day-per-week training programs if the time is available. Our summer and off-season programs for our higher-level athletes tend to be four-day programs. I also believe program design is easiest and most efficient in a four-day program.

Four-Day Training Programs

Training four times a week is the gold standard for training programs in a perfect world. The following chart takes the components discussed in chapter 3 and demonstrates how these quantities fit into a four-day workout.

The tables on the following pages are the key to this entire book. Once you understand the concept, the table is like a "fill in the blank" template for programming workouts.

Strength and Conditioning Coaching

DAY 1	DAY 2	DAY 3	DAY 4
Warm-Up, Mobility, Speed, and Plyometrics (45 minutes)			
Foam Roll	Foam Roll	Foam Roll	Foam Roll
Static Stretch	Static Stretch	Static Stretch	Static Stretch
Mobility/Activation	Mobility/Activation	Mobility/Activation	Mobility/Activation
Warm-Up Linear	Warm-Up Multi-Direction	Warm-Up Linear	Warm-Up Multi-Direction
Linear Plyos Chest Pass Linear Sprints	Lateral Plyos Rotary/Overhead Med Ball	Linear Plyos Chest Pass Linear Sprints	Lateral Plyos Rotary/Overhead Med Ball
Timed 10s on Days 1 and 3			
Power and Strength Development (35–45 minutes)			

PAIR 1	PAIR 1	PAIR 1	PAIR 1
Explosive/Olympic Lifts	Hip Dominant (Trap Bar)	Explosive/Olympic Lifts	Knee Dominant (Unilateral)
Core: Anti-Rotation (Chop)	Core: Anti-Lateral	Core: Anti-Rotation (Lift)	Core: Anti-Lateral
	Vertical Pull		Horizontal Pull

PAIR 2	PAIR 2	PAIR 2	PAIR 2
Horizontal Press (Bench Press)	Knee Dominant (Unilateral)	Horizontal Press (Incline or Close Grip Bench)	Hip Dominant (Unilateral)
Stretch: Upper	Horizontal Pull	Stretch: Upper	Vertical Pull

PAIR 2	PAIR 2	TRI-SET 1	TRI-SET 1
Vertical Press	Hip Dominant (Slide Board Lunge, Ham Iso, Slide Board Leg Curl)	Push-Up Variation	Hip Dominant (Slide Board Lunge, Ham Iso, Slide Board Leg Curl)
Hip Rehab Specialty Work	Core: Anti-Extension	Rotary or Rehab Specialty Work	Core: Anti-Extension

Strength and Conditioning Coaching

On days one and three, the focus is on power development through Olympic lifting or some type of weighted or resisted jump. This is the biggest change we've made in a decade from a strength and power training perspective. In order to get the amount of lower-body work I now feel is required, we're forced to move our Olympic movements to what's primarily an upper-body day.

This is a basic template for a healthy athlete, but not for *every* athlete. For athletes with injury problems who are unable to Olympic lift, we may substitute trap bar jumps, jump squats or jumps on the MVP shuttle. The important thing is to get some explosive resisted hip and knee extension, not to force everyone to Olympic lift.

Note that Olympic movements aren't paired with other strength exercises. Exercises with a high neural and technical demand shouldn't be paired with another physically demanding exercise. The explosive, total-body nature of these exercises isn't conducive to this. In our setting, we're using our diagonal patterns and/or rotary stability exercises during the time between explosive sets.

Days two and four of the strength and power program consists of pairs of major multi-joint exercises sometimes complemented by a core exercise or a mobility drill to form a tri-set.

Without using a tri-set concept, it's difficult to address all the categories that must be included in a program. Although this is a compromise, our structure keeps the workout to approximately an hour. Research indicates that strength workouts longer than that can result in significant cortisol build-up.

Moving explosive lifts to our upper-body day also allows a third pair of exercises to be added to the workouts on days two and four.

The third section of the program varies depending on the specific phase of the program, but it generally includes an overhead or vertical press, a rotary exercise and some type of rehabilitative or specialty work for the hips or shoulders. On days two and four, we may add some type of additional posterior-chain work.

Three-Day Workout Programs

DAY 1	DAY 2	DAY 3
Movement Skill and Conditioning (1 hour)		
For warm-up, speed development, plyometrics conditioning, the days can be alternated linear–lateral–linear in the first week and lateral–linear–lateral in the second week. This allows three linear workouts every two weeks and three multi-directional workouts every two weeks.		
Explosive/Olympic	Explosive/Olympic	Explosive/Olympic
Chop Progression	Lift Progression	Anti-Rotation

TRI-SET 1	TRI-SET 1	TRI-SET 1
Hip Dominant Double-Leg	Knee Dominant Unilateral	Knee Dominant Unilateral
Core: Anti-Extension	Core: Anti-Lateral Flexion	Core: Anti-Extension
Horizontal Press	Incline Press	Vertical Press
TRI-SET 2	**TRI-SET 2**	**TRI-SET 2**
Knee Dominant Single-Leg	Vertical Press	Horizontal Press
Vertical Pull	Horizontal Pull	Horizontal Pull
Hip Dominant Straight-Leg	Hip Dominant Bent-Leg	Rotary or Rehab

Three-day workouts follow a few different patterns depending on the situation. If the workout is a Monday–Wednesday–Friday pattern, the workout is a total-body workout each day.

This is the pattern illustrated in the sample program and worksheet.

In a school setting, three-day programs can also be done Monday–Tuesday–Thursday or Tuesday–Thursday–Friday to increase time utilization in the weightroom. The difference here is that you'd have two consecutive days and one non-consecutive day. The two consecutive days are performed like the four-day split (use the four-day plan) with the third, non-consecutive day being a total-body workout. In other words, for a Monday–Tuesday–Thursday program, you'd use days one and two from the four-day program and on Thursday, you'd plan a total-body workout.

Three-day programs include numerous compromises. It's no longer possible to work each movement pattern two times during a week. Vertical pressing and some upper pulling patterns might only be done once per week, while some hip-dominant exercises and horizontal pressing may be done twice.

If you fill in the blocks with the exercises of your choosing for a three-day program, you have 25% fewer blocks to complete than in a four-day program. As a result, compromises must be made, and the overall effectiveness of the workout is decreased potentially by the same 25%.

Are three-day workouts inherently bad? No, but recognize that it's more difficult to put the pieces together in a three-day program. We have begun to experiment more with three-day programs with our collegiate athletes. There are some benefits to three-day programs from a speed perspective as sprints and sprint-related drills and exercises can be done three times per week on non-consecutive days. Three-day workouts also allow for slightly more lower-body variety if you utilize three non-consecutive total-body days.

Strength and Conditioning Coaching

Two-Day Workout Programs

SAMPLE TWO-DAY WORKOUT BREAKDOWN	
Warm-Up—combine linear and lateral concepts	
Linear Plyo Lateral Plyo	
Three Med Ball Throws—rotary, overhead, chest pass	
DAY 1	**DAY 2**
PAIR 1	**PAIR 1**
Explosive/Olympic Combo	Explosive/Olympic Combo
Diagonal Core (Chop/Lift)	Diagonal Core (Chop/Lift)
PAIR 2	**PAIR 2**
Hip-Dominant Double-Leg	Knee-Dominant Single-Leg
Horizontal Supine Press	Incline Press/Close-Grip Bench
TRI-SET 3	**TRI-SET 3**
Vertical Pull	Horizontal Pull
Knee-Dominant Single-Leg	Hip-Dominant Straight-Leg
Core/Rotary/Rehab	Core/Rotary/Rehab

Two-day workouts force us to modify some of the initial recommendations. All of the necessary exercise categories will be addressed once in a two-day program. Each day features a knee-dominant exercise, a hip-dominant exercise, a pushing exercise and a pulling exercise.

Two-day programs in our context should be reserved for in-season lifting or for high school athletes who are only off-season in the summer. Two-day programs are also great for endurance athletes who don't have the time to strength train three or four times per week.

Using the Yessis 1 x 20?

For those unfamiliar, Dr. Michael Yessis wrote an entire book on the 1 x 20 idea. Matt Thome has also written excellent articles on the concept.

I'll summarize as best I can from my readings. Basically, athletes perform one set of 20 reps for 15–20 different exercises.

The program generally proceeds from multi-joint exercises to single-joint exercises and, as described in the book, features quite a few simple, single-joint exercises we'd never use at MBSC.

However, that doesn't take away from the concept of a higher-volume, lower-intensity phase as a change-up. As with any programming concept, feel free to interpret the idea in your own environment.

For us at MBSC, I like the 1 x 20 as a change-up for athletes we work with year-round. In a 12-week off-season program, 1 x 20 isn't a good fit, but for year-round athletes, it can be a great change of pace.

First, let me say that 1 x 20 is a bit of a misnomer, at least according to what I've read. Athletes only do 1 x 20 in week one of the program, and over a three-week phase, the program is generally 20–14–10 or 20–14–8. For the percentage readers (and for simplicity's sake, I am one), we did 60% in week one, 68% in week two and 78% in week three. I know this isn't perfect, but trust me and try it.

We also had to figure out how an idea like 1 x 20 fits for power exercises such as Olympic lifts where we'd never do 20 reps for bodyweight exercises like chin-ups and for unilateral exercises.

Our solutions were as follows:

Olympic Lifts—Instead of 1 x 20, we start with 4 x 5 for a total of 20 reps of, for example, hang clean.

Chin-Ups—The goal is 20 reps in as few sets as possible. We push for a max set on set one and then fill in the rest.

Unilateral Exercises—For unilateral exercises, we'll do 10 reps on each side in phase one. I'm just not a fan of 20 reps for unilateral exercises. From both a time and technique standpoint, sets of 20 on each side can be a challenge.

In-Season Training Specifics

I get lots of questions about in-season training. The requests always start with, "I need an in-season training program for _____." You can add your sport in the blank.

Let's start with one of my favorite quotes:

"Your sport isn't different; you just think it is."

I first heard those words spoken by Marco Cardinale, former Head of Sports Science and Research for the British Olympic Association. He was discussing how every sport coach he encountered in preparation for the London Olympics thought their sport needed a specific program.

Sport-specific programs are at best an 80/20 proposition. Eighty percent of programs will be the same, while 20 percent may be specific to the sport. I even think it's more like 90/10.

The truth is all in-season programs look amazingly similar. Programs tend to be two days a week, with low-volume basic lifts and no conditioning.

With in-season strength training the emphasis is on getting in and getting out. Players tend to be tired and potentially uninterested. I liken in-season training to trips to the dentist. People don't like them but view them as a necessary evil that prevents problems down the road.

There might be subtle differences based on the sport, but in-season training is really basic *The Slight Edge* stuff.

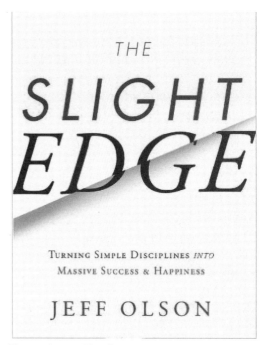

Figure 10.1—The Slight Edge, a "must read."

Jeff Olson, the author of the book *The Slight Edge*, describes things simply:

Number 1—Show up. Eighty percent of success is showing up.

Number 2—Be consistent. Keep showing up.

Number 3—Build a good attitude and enjoy showing up.

Number 4—Be committed for a long period of time. Just keep showing up and show up happy.

Number 5—Have faith and a burning desire.

Number 6—Be willing to pay the price.

Number 7—Practice slight-edge integrity. What do you do when no one is watching?

This is what in-season training is all about. Show up, and show up consistently. Don't miss; don't skip; don't make excuses.

Once you get that part established, the rest is simple. Push, pull, legs, core—low-volume high-intensity work. One or two sets are all you need after the warm-up sets.

I like to say, *"The best way to get stronger is not to get weaker."*

That's the key to in-season work. Don't go backward if you're strong; get stronger in season if you're a beginner.

Strength and Conditioning Coaching

A few tips:

Consistency is key—have we said that? One reason it's so important to be consistent is that athletes hate to be sore in-season. If you skip a workout or worse yet, skip lower body (a huge mistake), players are sore for a few days. Being sore for a few days can ruin an in-season program. No one wants to be sore before a game.

If your athletes play only on weekends, lift heavy early in the week. I know it may seem counterproductive, but players want to feel fresh come game time.

Don't go below five reps for lower body. Think risk–reward or risk–benefit. The risk of a heavy low-rep set just isn't worth it. Want to get coaches to jump off the in-season lifting bandwagon? Get a player hurt in the weightroom.

When in doubt, reread Olson's list. Thinking about cancelling a workout because the players are tired? Don't do it. *The Slight Edge* point two is consistency. Week off? Nope, consistency. The key to in-season training is showing up.

I am 100% convinced success in terms of wins and losses can be impacted by a good, consistent in-season program.

And keep reminding yourself that something is better than nothing! Get it done. If players are genuinely tired, do a quick "set of 10" workout. Pick exercises like single-leg squats and chin-ups where 10 reps provide a pretty good stimulus. Just run though a push–pull–legs–core single-set circuit, but don't *not* lift. Precede this with an extra-long foam roll, stretch and dynamic warm-up, and finish with some stretching. Your athletes will thank you.

Training Consecutive Days?

I've always recommended two-day-per-week in-season programs. One coach took this to mean it would be okay to train two days, using consecutive days to do an upper-lower split. This, in my mind, defeats the purpose.

Let me clear something up: In-season training should consist of two *non-consecutive* total-body workouts. Doing a split routine is actually like training once, not twice.

Sets and Reps

Sets and reps choices are easy. I like to undulate the reps every three weeks, and I like to keep sets low. Three sets of an exercise would be very high volume for us in-season. Most often, we do one or two sets. We rarely go beyond 10 reps in-season. We also rarely do fewer than three reps.

For power exercises, we simply alternate between three sets of three and three sets of five. For strength exercises, we use 2 x 5, 2 x 8 or 2 x 10. Most assistance-type exercises are done for two sets of 10 throughout the in-season period.

Ladder, Plyos or Agilities

Another question that frequently comes up is, "What about ladder work, agility or plyos?" The in-season program is primarily a strength program. If we lift post-practice, we don't do any pre-workout preparatory things. We come off the field, pick up our sheets and begin lifting. If we lift prior to practice, we follow our normal pre-practice routine of foam rolling, static stretching and dynamic warm-ups. However, we will do a bit of speed and power in-season, particularly if we lift before practice, hitting one or two Flying 10-yard sprints and 15 to 30 plyo reps. We'd continue to do this in the weightroom if I couldn't sell the sport coach on adding these on the field or the ice.

In-Season Training for American Football

Football can be a long season, with college seasons often spanning more than five months. The longer the season, the more important the in-season period becomes.

One program I've always loved for in-season athletes—and I think I'd be using this in every sport if I was a college strength coach—was referred to as the "Russian peaking cycle." Just the name is enough to get geeky strength coaches excited.

The Russian peaking cycle was first introduced to me through an article by Dr. Fred Hatfield describing a powerlifting routine. For those who aren't strength and conditioning historians, Hatfield, known as "Dr.

Squat," was the world record holder in the squat in weight classes from 181 to 276. Many of his books and articles are long since lost, but the concept has remained in my head for decades. I'm not even sure about the name, but I guess in the 1980s, "Russian" already had a secretive tone to it.

The current copy of the routine I looked at to verify my memory was provided on the website *liftvault.com*. Take a look.[14]

In-season training for football presents interesting issues. It's essential that a football player maintains or increases strength during the in-season period. Yet players must do this while putting the body through the extreme stresses of physical contact on an almost daily basis.

These two processes seem to be mutually exclusive. Dealing with the soreness produced by the first few weeks of contact while at the same time beginning an in-season program to maintain (or even improve in the case of freshmen and redshirts), strength gains can seem like an impossibility.

The solution I found most effective was the modified Russian peaking cycle. The key to this is the athlete is only asked to lift 80 percent of the 1RM for sets of two reps. This is well below the expected seven or eight reps at 80%, and allows the players to "feel" a moderately heavy weight.

For the next four weeks (weeks two to five), the load doesn't increase, and we simply ask for one additional rep per week, ending with 80% for six reps. This is very similar to the 5–6–7–8–9 for kids idea in chapter 9. Initially, the loads are well below the athlete's actual capability, and as a result, very achievable.

In weeks six to 10, the load is increased by 2.5% per week while the reps are decreased by one per week. The end result is athletes performing singles over 90% in week 10.

If they can simply stay with the program, they'll have maintained a minimum of 90% of their preseason strength. This is done without ever doing more than six reps per set and can be done with starters for as little as one heavy set per week.

A little can go a long way in-season.

The following can be used for the trap bar deadlift, bench press, hang clean or any exercise you view as a primary lift.

The Russian Peaking Cycle
(Modified for In-Season)

Week 1

80% x 2 x 2

Week 2

80% x 3 x 2

Week 3

80% x 4 x 2

Week 4

80% x 5 x 2

Week 5

80% x 6 x 2

Week 6

82.5% x 5 x 2

Week 7

85% x 4 x 2

Week 8

87.5% x 3 x 3

Week 9

90% x 2 x 3

Week 10

92.5% x 1 x 3

*The original called for up to six sets.

In-Season Training for Soccer and Field Hockey

As previously mentioned, in-season strength training for any sport really shouldn't vary greatly. The goals of all in-season programs are nearly identical.

One big goal is to, at a minimum, maintain strength and power for upperclassmen, and ideally improve strength and power for freshmen and redshirts.

The information on in-season training for football highlights a strength cycle that might be useful for any sport in-season. The only difference between in-season training for football and

---

14   https://liftvault.com/programs/powerlifting/fred-hatfields-peaking-program-spreadsheet/#:~:text=Developed%20by%20Fred%20Hatfield%20%28aka%20Dr.%20Squat%29%2C%20this,period%20half%20way%20through%20the%20program%20for%20recovery
Bobbert M. (1990) Drop jumping as a training method for jumping ability. Sports Medicine 9, 7-22 [PubMed] [Google Scholar]

in-season training in another sport is that football coaches and football strength coaches place a great emphasis on in-season strength training. This shouldn't be unique and in fact, should be the same for every sport.

In sports like field hockey and soccer, good consistent training during the in-season period will form the backbone of the long-term success of both the strength program and of the entire sports program. Remember,

"The best way to get stronger is to not get weaker."
~ Michael Boyle

Bottom line, it's much easier to get stronger in the off-season when we maintain strength during the season. It's a waste of valuable training time to spend the off-season regaining lost strength. Whether at the high school or collegiate level, the training program should be viewed as a four-year process. In an ideal world, training will be a continual upward progression of strength, power and speed every year.

I've used some of the same keys from the football section because the body isn't different for different sports. The only thing that's different is the coach's perception.

Keys to In-Season Programming

Get frequent workouts (realistically two per week) with higher intensities but lower volumes. Intensity is the key to training, not volume, and this applies even more in-season. Never skip an in-season workout. A 15-minute, one-set workout is far better in the long run than a missed day.

Work lower-body strength and power in-season. Don't try to "save the legs." If you save them in September, they'll fail you in November. See number one again: high intensity, low volume. One or two sets of an Olympic lift and one or two sets of a squat or deadlift variation go a long way.

Only listen to "workers" not "whiners." As a general rule, I say, "Don't let the inmates run the asylum." Most athletes don't

like in-season lifting. It's like going to the dentist, necessary and often painful. Take my advice: Most young people don't know what's good for them and will usually take the path of least resistance. Give them no optional workouts, no choices of lifts and allow no phantom injuries that mean they can't work the lower body.

I came up with a simple solution to the injury question. You have to convince your sport coaches that if athletes are too injured to lift, they're too injured to play. You'll be amazed how fast kids get healthy. Our policy is that if the "injured" athletes didn't talk to the trainer and arrange treatment, they aren't actually hurt.

Field Hockey Specific Issues—Some may consider this sexist, but I'm going to say it anyway: Most of the female athletes I've worked with, and nearly every field hockey player, find muscular legs unattractive. Muscular legs, wanted or not, are a necessary evil in sports. One way to compromise is to include more hip-dominant and less knee-dominant work, like maybe single-leg squats once a week and either trap bar deadlifts and single-leg SLDLs or slide board lunges the other day. This means prioritizing glutes and hamstrings over quads.

This might get me in trouble too, but the reality is that most women fear becoming too muscular. Whether it's a realistic fear doesn't matter. So, focus on strength not volume, and prioritize the posterior chain.

Soccer Specific Issues—Male soccer players, in my experience, have no problem working on the upper body, but will avoid leg work like the plague. Don't allow a male soccer player to go near a bench or a curl bar until the explosive work and lower-body work is finished. Most male high school soccer players spend all their weightroom time working on muscles that have little value in soccer. For women, follow the lower-body recommendations for field hockey.

Bottom line: Do quick workouts with an emphasis on higher intensity (heavier weight) and lower body and lower volume (fewer sets). Give them no choices. Make them do the work.

CHAPTER 11
SPEED DEVELOPMENT

First off, I want to thank Stu McMillan from Altis for reading parts of this chapter and for his objective feedback and critique. This book got better thanks to Stu.

Please understand, if you're coaching elite track and field athletes—elite meaning at least national caliber—this chapter wasn't written for you. This chapter was written for high school and college strength coaches who might previously have been testing speed two or three times a year, or sadly, less.

I love track coaches. I learn from track coaches, but just like my athletes aren't powerlifters or Olympic lifters, they aren't track athletes either. We can modify the Denis Logan quote to:

"We want great athletes who are good sprinters."

In our setting, we don't have all day to work on speed or to run a track practice. We need to be efficient and effective.

Imagine if I said I had a magic exercise. Velocity is in the eight-meters-per-second range. You can max in the exercise six to eight times per week at 97–100% safely for months on end, and the exercise will produce rapid improvement. Well, I have that exercise, and it's called the Flying 10. Yes, a timed 10-yard sprint done with a "fly-in" phase of between 5 and 20 yards.

Player: "Coach, I need to get faster."
Coach: "Okay, how fast are you?"
Player: "I'm not sure. I haven't been timed."
Coach: "Then how do you know you're slow?"
Player: "I just know."

This scenario or a similar one plays out innumerable times a year all over the world. Everyone wants to get faster, even fast athletes. Sadly, most people don't even know how fast they are or, more likely, aren't.

Worse yet, many athletes think they're fast. Everybody's fast until the timer comes out. Trust me, 4.4s are rare and a 4.2 is like a unicorn.

This chart, provided by Coach Joe Stokowski of Pepperell High School in Georgia, provides a sobering look at how fast someone needs to be to run a 4.4 40.

The fastest athlete we've seen (through our Flying 10s) turned out to be a 4.55 40. To run a 4.2, he'd need to run .90 for 10 yards with a 20-yard fly-in—see the intersection of 4.2 and 2030 below. Our fastest athlete so far was .96.

Just FYI, 1020 is the Flying 10 time from 10 yards to 20 yards. This means the "fly-in" is 10 yards. 2030 means the fly-in is now 20 yards.

40 YARD	010	1020	2030	3040
4.10	1.42	0.98	0.88	0.82
4.15	1.44	0.99	0.89	0.83
4.20	1.46	1.00	0.90	0.84
4.25	1.48	1.01	0.91	0.85
4.30	1.50	1.02	0.92	0.86
4.35	1.52	1.03	0.93	0.87
4.40	1.54	1.04	0.94	0.88
4.45	1.56	1.05	0.95	0.89
4.50	1.58	1.06	0.96	0.90

40 YARD	010	1020	2030	3040
4.55	1.60	1.07	0.97	0.91
4.60	1.62	1.08	0.98	0.92
4.65	1.64	1.09	0.99	0.93
4.70	1.65	1.10	1.00	0.95
4.75	1.67	1.11	1.01	0.96
4.80	1.68	1.12	1.02	0.98
4.85	1.70	1.13	1.03	0.99
4.90	1.71	1.14	1.04	1.01
4.95	1.73	1.15	1.05	1.02
5.00	1.74	1.16	1.06	1.04
5.05	1.76	1.17	1.07	1.05
5.10	1.77	1.18	1.08	1.07
5.15	1.79	1.19	1.09	1.08
5.20	1.80	1.20	1.10	1.10
5.25	1.82	1.21	1.11	1.11
5.30	1.83	1.22	1.12	1.13
5.35	1.85	1.23	1.13	1.14

Acceleration or Top Speed

I've made a few bad assumptions about speed training in my career. The first assumption was that sport was just about acceleration, not speed. I've said and written this statement numerous times. The truth is I was at best about half right.

Most sport situations involve sprints of 10 yards or less. Most often, these sprints are started from a walk, a jog or from standing. This is clearly an acceleration scenario. I always loved using the 0–60 example with cars. With a car, 0–60 tells you about the car's "pick up."

But, ask yourself this: What's the 0–60 capability of a car that only goes 55? Therein lies failing number one—ignoring max speed. Increasing max speed will also increase acceleration capability. You can't go 0–60 if your max speed is 55!

My Epiphany

If you aren't timing your athletes on a regular basis, which we now do twice a week, you aren't doing speed training. Everyone wants their athletes to be faster; however, most coaches can't get out of their own way when it comes to developing speed.

Author's note: Until four years ago, I was one of those coaches.

As Dan Pfaff has famously said:

"Strength coaches have a PhD in the weight-room, but an elementary school level of education on sprinting."

Many coaches see our fascination with timing as evidence of my elementary school education in speed. I beg to differ. The difference with me is that I know my "students." I know what they need and, most importantly, I know how long "class" is.

In our pursuit of speed, we strength coaches run into a few problems.

Problem One

We desperately want to believe we can develop speed in the weightroom without actually sprinting. Most strength coaches view sprinting as a test to be done a few times a year, instead of as a training tool to be used frequently but judiciously.

As you evaluate your current speed improvement strategy, ask yourself these three questions:

1—Do my athletes consistently run fast in training?
2—Do they run fast twice every week year-round?
3—How do I know they're running fast?

The third question is the key. If you don't time your athletes, you don't know if they're running fast. You may think they're running fast, but are they? These aren't track athletes and there won't be meets to base things off.

When athletes lift, it's easy to look at the weight on the bar and make a simple judgment. With untimed "speed" work, it's not so easy.

Speed development goes back to the old Peter Drucker quote:

"What gets measured gets managed."

Or as Tony Holler says, "Record, rank, publish." This leads us to problem number two.

Problem Two

Strength coaches say they want to develop speed, but they rarely test speed and probably don't even train it. Doing technical sprint drills isn't speed training; it's the warm-up for speed training. Working on sprint mechanics isn't speed training; it's also a warm-up. Sprinting is speed training. You can't simply test speed twice a year and have it be a pass or fail proposition. You also can't just do a bunch of drills and think you're building a speed program.

The best analogy I read was in the book *Most Likely to Succeed*. The authors spoke about how bike riding might be taught in school.

"It would start by students learning all of the parts of the bike. I'm not sure how useful that information has ever been to me in my bike riding history, but from there, they might learn the history of bikes, learn the physics of how the gears and chain work to propel the bike,

might watch other people riding a bike, and test the effectiveness of various bikes. In no part of this learning would anyone actually be riding a bike."

This is how I view most speed training programs. As, Bs, dribbles…etc…etc., but no timed sprints. The parts don't really matter; riding the bike is what matters. What matters for us is how fast athletes get from A to B.

I've seen so much time wasted turning people into pretty runners through lots of drills. Guess what? Lots of them are "pretty slow." We're constantly seeing our videos of fast people being critiqued for not being pretty, but they *are* pretty fast.

The problem, as I've already stated, is that most coaches view timed sprinting as a test. This test is done perhaps two or three times per year and that day and the days leading up to it are generally filled with anxiety and trepidation.

Will my athletes improve?

Did my "speed" program work?

Will anyone get injured?

A test-day hamstring pull in this situation is almost a given. It's like athletes can feel your anxiety, and they tighten up too.

The real key to speed improvement is to get coaches to reorient their lens and see sprinting not as a test, but as a training tool that needs to be used twice a week. In order to use the tool properly, you need to time your athletes!

When people want to get faster, the first thing we need to know is how fast they are now. We need a "before." It's not how fast they think they are. We need good, solid, valid and reliable data. But then, problem number three might be the biggest impediment to speed development.

Problem Three

For years—decades really—strength coaches have deluded themselves into believing they can develop speed in the weightroom. It's amazing that strength coaches can run a primarily vertical weightroom program and expect significant horizontal changes.

(*Yes, I understand there's a vertical component to speed, but for most of us, there's no horizontal component in the weightroom. Thanks, Stu McMillan, for calling me out on this oversimplification.*)

Don't get me wrong, I'm a huge weightroom person, but as strength coaches, we've overvalued weightroom strength as a tool to develop speed. We still need to lift for "armor building," injury prevention and a host of other reasons, but I'm no longer sure how much effect conventional weightroom strength has on speed once we get past the intermediate level.

But Increased Mass Makes for Greater Collisions?

As I said, I'm a huge weightroom proponent. Bigger athletes generally tend to be better. If we can maintain speed while increasing mass, we improve "sprint momentum."

My man Bryan Mann (pun intended) sent me this formula. I was going to dub this "The Mann Sprint Momentum Formula" until Coach Dan Baker told me he thought of it first. The formula shows a big reason the weightroom is so important in any sport involving body contact.

Sprint Momentum = BW in KGs x 10-yard time in meters/sec

So: (BW/2.2) x (9.14/10-yard time)

In contact sports, this means we need to work on both sides of the equation. Track isn't a contact sport. In any body contact sport, additional body mass without speed loss produces greater forces.

We need to work on both sides of this, not just the bodyweight side. Maintaining speed while increasing mass matters.

If conventional strength training developed speed the way many strength coaches would like to believe it does, we'd have lots of powerlifters running in track meets and winning Olympic medals...but we don't.

Record, Rank, Publish?

A few years ago, Coach Tony Holler caused me to make the single biggest change in our programming in decades. Tony's "Record, Rank and Publish" article made me rethink what we were doing for speed development. And when I say rethink, we're talking about a major change in thought process and a major change in our programming.

Like many coaches, we at MBSC thought we were doing a pretty good job with our speed training. We lifted, did our plyos and "ran sprints." However, we were making a few critical mistakes.

Mistake 1—Most lifting is vertical and bilateral, but speed has both vertical and horizontal components and is obviously unilateral. Let's face it, Olympic lifts, squats and deadlifts are done up and down, not forward. And yes, they're going to help, but our athletes need unilateral and horizontal work.

Mistake 2—In addition, most of our plyos were also vertical or at least more vertically oriented. We didn't do enough horizontal or unilateral plyometric work. Thanks to Rob Assise for driving that one home.

Mistake 3—This was the biggest one: Our sprints weren't actually sprints. I think we did some fast running, but I'm not sure how many athletes actually sprinted.

I have to digress for a minute and mention that Coach Steve Bunker, who runs our Middleton facility, had been advocating doing timed 10s for years. I pushed back against timed sprints (and Coach Bunker) for two really bad reasons:

1—Laziness. Setting up timers every day, changing batteries, dealing with technical difficulties and more just seemed like too much work. Why not just run five or six untimed sprints and be done? I thought timing just added an unnecessary layer of complexity.

2—Fear. Yes, fear. Timing made me think of hamstring pulls. I hate injuries.

But, what's the *Animal House* line? To paraphrase, "Dumb and lazy is no way to go through life."

The bottom line is, if you aren't timing, you can't be sure you're sprinting. I know this may give some people pause, but think about it this way: For running to be considered "speed work," you need to run at 90% of max speed or faster for a given distance. Some might even say 95%.

Logically, if we don't know the speed over a given distance, how we can we determine if we've passed the 90% threshold? Ninety percent of what?

If I don't know how fast you can run 10 yards, how can I know what 90% of that time is? Ten yards takes about 1.2 to 1.5 seconds on average. That means anything over 1.65 isn't really speed work.

In my first 38 years, we ran a lot, but I'm not sure how much actual speed work we did. The devil is in the details, as they say. One thing I know is that the "eye test" doesn't work. Timing creates intent and when done properly, it creates intrinsic competition. The timer also encourages self-organization without the fear of "losing."

Note: We never race. This eliminates a potentially powerful and negative extrinsic variable—an opponent in a race. In addition, as Tony Holler loves to say, "Getting beat is not performance enhancing."

So, we've talked a lot about problems and mistakes. How about a few potential solutions?

Proposed Solution One: Timing 10-Yard Dashes

I've started to refer to sprinting as "real velocity-based training." Why try to squat fast when running fast is safer and easier to do?

Fast squats are less than two meters per second. Average sprinting is eight meters per second. If we do the math from a velocity-based standpoint, are sprints four times better than squats?

We now time a specific and progressive variation of a 10-yard sprint twice per week following what I call "Tony's Rules."

Tony's Rule #1—One athlete at a time. Coaches love competition, but kids get tight when they compete. They worry too much about the opponent and not enough about themselves. Competition in sprinting is one person against his or her best time. Their goal is to beat their time, not someone else's. Trust me, kids will compete against each other's times anyway. Don't line up for races unless you're comfortable with injuries.

Tony's Rule #2—Two or three sprints a day, no more. More isn't better. We've occasionally run four sprints, but have never done five. That means we run somewhere between a low of four and a high of eight sprints per week.

We also follow "Mike's Rules!"

Mike's Rule #1—We're adamant about the question "*Does it hurt?*"

I get asked exercise questions all the time. I've worked with athletes in almost every major sport who were told they were "all done" by a doctor or a trainer. Because people know my background, they often ask for advice on dealing with injuries or on selecting exercises.

Unfortunately, most of the time, they ignore the advice because the advice doesn't contain the answer they want. They say something like, "It only hurts when I run." I answer, "Don't run."

A famous coach I know once told me, "People don't look for advice. They look for agreement or consensus. If you don't tell them what they want to hear, they simply ask someone else." His advice was to stop wasting my time giving advice.

Well, here I go again wasting time.

Before you work with injured athletes, imagine you have an injury and are wondering whether a certain exercise is appropriate, and ask yourself a simple question: "Does it hurt?"

The question of "Does it hurt?" can only be answered with a yes or no. If the answer is yes, your athlete isn't ready for that exercise, no matter how much you like the exercise or want to use it. Simple, right? Not really.

I tell everyone I speak with that any equivocation is a yes. Responses like, "After I warm up, it goes away" are yes answers. It's amazing how many times I've asked people this simple question only to have them dance around it—they dance around it because they don't like my answer. They want to know things like, "What about the magic cure no one has told me about?" or "What about a secret exercise?"

I have another saying I like: "The secret is there is no secret." Another wise man, Ben Franklin I think it was, said, "Common sense is not so common."

If your athlete is injured, use your common sense. Exercise shouldn't cause pain. This seems simple, but exercisers, especially athletes, ignore and rationalize pain all the time.

Discomfort is common at the end of a set of a strength exercise or at the end of an intense cardiovascular workout. The discomfort of delayed onset muscle soreness often occurs the two days following an intense session. This is normal. This discomfort should only last two days and should be limited to the muscles, not the joints or tendons.

Pain at the onset of an exercise is neither normal nor healthy, and is indicative of a problem.

Progression in any strength exercise should be based on a full, pain-free range of motion that produces muscle soreness without joint soreness. If you need to change or reduce the range of motion, it's a problem.

Progression in cardiovascular exercise should also be pain-free and should follow the 10% rule. Don't increase time or distance more than 10% from one session to the next.

I've used these simple rules in all of my strength and conditioning programs and have been able to keep literally thousands of athletes healthy. I'm sure the same concepts will help you with yours.

We're constantly reminding our athletes not to sprint if they don't feel "perfect." I know this sounds like common sense, but you'll be surprised by how many athletes will tell you that they sprinted in spite of being sore…and now they feel worse.

I frequently hear, "*I felt a little something on the one before.*" That drives me nuts. Teach your kids to respect their bodies. Full-speed sprinting can and will hurt your trainees when done in a less-than-perfect state.

Another thought: No one should be made fun of or belittled for not running sprints. Sore from practice the night before? No sprints. Tournament over the weekend and feeling a little tight? No sprints. Our goal is to get faster, not hurt. Nothing disrupts training and progress like an injury.

A suggestion from Dan Pfaff: Substitute a few bike sprints for athletes who can't sprint that day. We replace our timed 10s with four 10-second bike sprints on days people are sore. This does two things. First, it discourages them from simple laziness because the bike sprints are harder than the Flying 10s. Second, it gives us a safe speed emphasis.

And yes, I know 10 seconds is too long. However, we discovered five-second bike sprints are a great way to break bikes.

Proposed Solution Two: Do More Horizontal Speed and Power Work

We now include sled marches as a strength exercise and sled sprints as a power exercise.

Think of the sled push as a standing closed-chain horizontal leg press. Think of sled sprints as horizontal Olympic lifts. We don't eliminate our conventional vertical strength training because this is still important; however, we make a point to better address the horizontal component.

In addition, we're power skipping more. I've never been a bounding fan because average athletes are poor bounders, but everyone can power skip. Thanks again to Rob Assise for really driving this home for me.

Also, we try to prioritize unilateral plyos over bilateral, meaning fewer hurdle jumps (two legs) and more hurdle hops (one leg).

Note: Vertical lower-body strength doesn't translate directly to speed as many strength coaches would like us to believe. Any student of speed will tell you most of the commonly used exercises for speed development work hip extension, but the force is primarily directed in a vertical direction. The ability to apply force to the ground and create forward movement can only occur when the foot is placed under the center of mass and the push is directed back.

Although squats and other lower-body movements will train the muscles involved in sprinting, the training isn't specific to the actions of acceleration or top speed. This may be one reason we see a higher correlation to vertical jump improvement than to speed improvement through conventional strength training. This is something we saw for years, but sadly didn't react to. It wasn't unusual for us to see 10–20% increases in vertical jump scores with very little change in speed.

What's a Good Time?

"What's a good time?" is a question I hear all the time. My answer is always, "For whom?" and then, "What's the fly-in?"

I can provide times for elite professional hockey players, elite women's hockey players (US Olympians and NWHL), elite college hockey players (NCAA Division 1 men's and women's) and high-end middle schoolers. I don't have quite enough data on high schoolers yet, but it's coming.

In order to even have the "What's a good time?" discussion, we need to establish a few parameters. Tony Holler's times for Flying 10s are taken in the 30–40-yard segment of a 40-yard dash. We'd refer to this as a 30-yard fly-in. To be clear, this means the last 10 yards of the 40-yard dash is recorded as the Flying 10 time.

As a result, we can't compare our 10-yard fly-in times to Tony's 30-yard fly-in times. The length of the fly-in will obviously influence the time. A longer fly-in will pretty consistently yield a lower time.

We've been doing 5-, 10-, 15- and 20-yard fly-ins. Every athlete gets faster as we add an additional five yards, up to 15 yards. With a 20-yard fly-in, we don't always see a change from the 15-yard fly-in. This may indicate team sport athletes are close to top speed by 25 yards.

The following is our progression.

Phase 1 is a 5-yard fly-in. This means twice per week we run a series of timed 10-yard dashes with a 5-yard fly-in.

All Flying 10s are recorded with an ArenaGear or Brower electronic timer. For Flying 10s, you'll need two sets of sensors.

Standing starts are a big key, as this eliminates the need to work on start technique. Coaches waste lots of time teaching and arguing about start technique, false steps and plyo steps when these have little relevance to sport performance.

As mentioned, we do two to four reps twice per week. The sprints are done after we've done our dynamic warm-up and after plyometrics and med ball throws. The warm-up may also include two to four reps through an acceleration ladder (think wickets, minus the wickets), two to four wicket runs or some combination.

We never run from a three- or four-point stance. The only people who might need a three-point stance are football linemen and those attending combines. A four-point stance or block start should be reserved for track and field. I'm embarrassed to think how much time I've wasted teaching starts to athletes who'll never be in a "hand on the ground position" in their sports. Understanding this allows us to get a more apples-to-apples comparison.

These are "good" times for a 5-yard fly-in.

NHL / Div I - 1.2-1.3 sec

Elite Female (USWNT) - 1.35-1.45 sec

High School Male - 1.2-1.3 sec

High School Female - 1.35-1.45 sec

Middle School Male- 1.35-1.45 sec

Middle School Female - 1.4-1.5 sec

How a Fly-In Affects Time

A 5-yard fly-in will lower the standing 10 time by about .1 seconds. This means a person who runs a 1.5 second standing 10 will run a 1.4 with a 5-yard fly-in. Going to a 10-yard fly-in will lower the time by an additional .1 seconds.

However, adding an additional 5 yards (a 15-yard fly-in) only drops the time by .05. As mentioned, moving to 20 yards lowered times by about .02, but in some cases not at all. As with everything we do, progression is key.

We work in three-week phases, so athletes will run 12–24 timed 10s in a phase. The progression is important because there's built-in progress based on the added fly-in distance—times get faster every phase, avoiding the feeling of plateaus. In addition, the total distance sprinted increases every phase.

Phase 2 is a 10-yard fly-in, again done twice per week. We stay with two to four timed reps per day for a total of six to eight sprints per week. Note that moving to a 10-yard fly-in increases the distance sprinted by 25 to 35%. Three 10-yard sprints with a 5-yard fly-in is 45 yards. The addition of a 10-yard fly-in ups the distance to 60 yards. We will usually do the first sprint at 5 yards and then two more at 10.

As previously mentioned, with a 10-yard fly-in, the time will drop by approximately .1 second.

Phase 3 is a 15-yard fly-in twice per week, two or three timed reps for a total of four to six (100–150 yards). Adding an additional 5 yards to the fly-in can again increase the distance sprinted by 25%.

With a 15-yard fly-in, the time will drop by .25 seconds from a standing 10. When we move to the 15-yard fly-in, the progression is usually a 5-yard fly-in on the first rep, 10 yards on the second and then one or two with 15.

Phase 4 (summer only) is a 20-yard fly-in twice per week, two or three timed reps for a total of four to six (120–180 yards). Please note that adding an additional 5 yards to the fly-in increases the distance sprinted by 25%.

The 20-yard fly-in only drops the time approximately .02, and in some cases, it doesn't drop at all.

This shows us that most team sport athletes are near max velocity by 25 yards (10-yard timed sprint with a 15-yard fly-in). If times drop, they drop by about .02. This would mean the 15-yard fly-in is about 98–100% of actual max velocity.

We follow the same progression of 5-10-15-20 for fly-ins. Rep 1 is from 5 yards, rep 2 from 10, rep 3 from 15 and a fourth and final rep from 20. In this case the athlete runs a 15-, a 20-, a 25- and a 30-yard sprint for a total distance of 90 yards. Again, on a good day, we might add an additional rep from 20 to hit 110 yards.

Reminder, moving from a 5-yard fly-in to a 10-yard fly-in drops the time by .1 second, moving to 15 drops the time by .15, but moving to 20 may be .02 or no change.

Top Flying 10 Times (20-yard fly-in)

NHL
.96-1.07 sec

Elite Women's Hockey (U.S. Olympians/NWHL)
1.07-1.19 sec

High School Male
1.0-1.02 sec

High School Female
1.10-1.12 sec

Middle School Male
1.1+-1.2+sec

Middle School Female
1.2+ sec

How Fast are Fast People? 10-Yard Fly Time to MPH

We hear a lot about athletes running greater than 20 MPH. However, in our speed development system, this is rare.

Due to facility constraints, we generally run our Flying 10s with either a 5-yard, 10-yard or 15-yard fly-in. Up to a point (and that point appears to be at least 20 yards), longer fly-ins tend to produce higher speeds.

The formula to convert fly-10 speeds to miles per hour is pretty straightforward:

$$20.45 \div 10y \text{ fly time} = mph$$

This means an athlete would have to run 1.02 to hit 20 MPH.

With a 15-yard fly-in, we've had only a few athletes do this. Jack Eichel, a former NHL Draft second overall pick, is one who consistently does it. I note this because 20 MPH appears to be world class with shorter fly-ins for non-track athletes.

Here's a quick chart:

1.0	*Flying 10 = 20.45 MPH*
1.1	*Flying 10 = 18.5 MPH*
1.2	*Flying 10 = 17 MPH*
1.3	*Flying 10 = 15.7 MPH*
1.4	*Flying 10 = 14.6 MPH*

Thanks again to Tony Holler for the conversion.

Self-Organization

"Self-organization, also called (in the social sciences) spontaneous order, is a process where some form of overall order arises from local interactions between parts of an initially disordered system. The process can be spontaneous when sufficient energy is available, not needing control by any external agent. It's often triggered by seemingly random fluctuations, amplified by positive feedback."
~ Wikipedia.org

Timed sprinting appears to be, at least to some degree, self-organizing. Athletes seem to get better at sprinting by sprinting, particularly in the early stages. The timer provides both positive and negative feedback as athletes experiment with different ideas.

This quote from Jorge Carvajal sums it up nicely:

"Sprinting teaches efficient running technique, and this, in essence, improves athleticism. That athleticism then develops a better athlete."

Note, "Sprinting teaches efficient running technique." Jorge didn't say, "Drills teach efficient running technique." He said sprinting.

Acceleration Versus Max Velocity in Team Sports

There's recently been lots of online back and forth between what I'll call the "max velocity crowd" and the "acceleration crowd." In general, the max velocity folks tend to be track coaches (generalizing a bit here), and the acceleration people tend to be working in team sports. Tony Holler says the "acceleration people" are weightroom people.

In the last couple of years, Tony's work has sparked a big interest in timing. This is good. However, as we tend to do in the strength and conditioning world, we've figured out how to argue about a topic most of us actually agree on.

Let's start with the idea that "timing is good." Tony's basic premise is that we can't get faster unless we know how fast we are. This is basically irrefutable—it's just logic. If I want to be faster than X, I need to know X.

Tony goes on to say we should also record the times and even rank the athletes fastest to slowest. I'm definitely into recording, but I am not sure ranking works in a non-team, private setting like ours at MBSC.

I think we can also agree on the idea that the best way to get fast is to run fast. If we accept the opinions of some of the experts, this means we need to run over 90% of our best time (X divided by .9).

However, in true "coach arguing" style, we've created something to argue about. The disagreement now seems not to be "should we time," but "what segment should we time?" And then, "How far should we run before we time it?"

In Tony's system, the Flying 10 time is taken from the 30–40 segment of a 40-yard dash. Tony's track athletes run lots of 40s. This means Tony's fly-in distance is 30 yards and also means that in Tony's view, they get a measure of maximum velocity.

Many in the sports performance world are timing Flying 10s, but with shorter fly-ins. MBSC would fall into that category. There are some pretty good reasons:

Facility logistics. Especially indoors in colder months, we have about 40 yards of total distance. This means we're limited to a Flying 10 with a 15-yard fly-in. There's no science here, just straight facility limits.

Injury concerns. There's some research indicating injuries increase as we move past 20 yards. Initially that limited us, but we've progressed outdoors to a 20-yard fly-in (30 yards) with no issues. Our lack of injuries may just be due to proper progression. Tony has experienced very few injuries with his 40-yard method. To contrast though, this means our longest sprint is 30 yards to Tony's 40.

Some coaches still subscribe to the idea that team sport athletes shouldn't run more than X number of yards and that sport is all about acceleration. Some coaches even argue that top speed or max velocity doesn't matter. More about that to follow.

Strangely, it seems if we don't select the 30–40 segment of the 40, we're labeled as "acceleration" and not "speed" coaches. Because our fly-in is only 20 yards, we're seen to be "neglecting" max velocity, and in effect, totally missing the boat.

Ken Clark's work has demonstrated that max velocity matters. In my mind, the goal is still the fastest possible Flying 10. We can look at this as time for a Flying 10 or as miles per hour.

However, acceleration is the most important quality in team sports—let's think of that as the 0–60 from the auto world. We have to consider the previously mentioned 0–60 capability of a car that only goes 55.

Top speed matters, even in acceleration. Ninety percent of 20 MPH is 18 MPH. Ninety percent of 18 miles per hour is 16.2 MPH. Math always wins.

The crux of the argument seems to be more about how far we need to run to hit max velocity. The argument the track people use is that world-class sprinters hit max velocity somewhere around 50–60 meters in a 100-meter race. In other words, they're accelerating for at least 50 meters.

Now, the fact that elite sprinters accelerate up to 50 meters has absolutely nothing to do with team sports. We've done extensive testing (1,000s of reps), and our athletes experience minimal change when we move from a 15- to 20-yard fly-in. The average change is about .01-.02, with many athletes showing no change at all. In simple terms, an athlete who is no longer accelerating has hit max velocity.

Poor Man's Sprint Training—or Feeding the Cats When You Have No Money

One question that comes up a lot is, "What do I do if I can't afford an electronic timer?" With the ArenaGear at under $700, I hope you'll prioritize and get a timer. However, we also have to be realistic and recognize that some programs just don't have the money.

Hand timing is a bad alternative; it's just not very accurate and with fly 10s, the margin of error is huge. Flying 10s take less than two seconds on average, so the error is probably double that of a 40.

Errors create all kinds of unrealistic expectations. If you mark it too fast, an athlete may never again get a personal record. Too slow and kids get discouraged that they aren't improving.

Although I really hate races, I may have a better solution. This idea is less than ideal and may not be as injury-free as using a timer. When kids compete against each other, we're adding a variable (an opponent) that may cause some people to effectively "try too hard" and potentially pull a muscle. Losing to the clock doesn't have the same stigma as losing to your best friend or your worst enemy and there's less of a sympathetic "fight or flight" response. I strongly prefer athletes run against the clock, but sometimes you need to bend the rules.

Strength and Conditioning Coaching

If you have to race, here's the "Feed the Poor Cats" program:

Weeks one to three, players sprint 15 yards twice per week, three times each for six sprints total. Remember, this is non-competitive for the first three weeks—no winners, no losers. It's just three sprints a day done after a dynamic warm-up.

I like to cue "push, push, push" to get athletes used to pushing hard against the ground.

In weeks four to six, you'll set up 15-yard one-on-one races. If these are lacrosse players, no sticks; if they're soccer players, no chasing balls, etc. Make the point be all about winning the race.

Try to create good pairs for competitive races, which will elicit 100% effort. Remember, only twice per week, three sprints each day, for a total of six sprints a week. This will cover the first six weeks.

Weeks seven to nine, players will progress to 20-yard races. Still do three sprints per day, two days a week. Weeks 10 to 12, move to 25 yards.

As a coach, you may think this isn't enough. Trust me, six maximal efforts a week is a lot. You'll also notice practice speed will increase. This isn't the only running they do, but it's maximal.

Remember: no improvisation, no skipped steps. Skipping steps is how kids get hurt.

And remember, make sure to perform a good dynamic warm-up prior to sprints. We follow our roll, stretch, dynamic warm-up process on every sprint day. We also do plyos and med ball work before sprints. Both serve as an additional warm-up.

Lastly: Never sprint sore. In almost every case, a player who sustains an injury no matter how minor during a sprint workout says afterward, "I felt a little something on the one before but kept going." Watch your athletes. Body language speaks volumes. Athletes stopping to stretch or massage a hamstring after a rep are saying "I felt that." Pull them out.

Sled Training

As often happens over my history, with sled training I was right, then wrong, then right again. In 2009, I wrote an article called "How to Use Sled Training to Drastically Improve Speed and Acceleration." In the article, I disagreed with mainstream views about pushing heavy sleds, running sled sprints and selecting sled loads. I advocated for heavy pushes and heavier sprints in spite of research showing the contrary.

Our empirical results showed us we were getting athletes faster—and we were pushing very heavy sleds slowly. I was right about almost everything in 2009, but still managed to drift from my own beliefs. Credit goes to Coach Cam Josse for pulling me back.

Over the last 20 to 30 years, numerous coaches and researchers have attempted to discredit the weighted sled as a tool for speed development, with many citing the potential for sled work to have a negative effect on top speed. However, in the past five years people in the research world such as JB Morin, Matt Cross and Pierre Samozino began to shed new light on an area many coaches empirically believed to be true. I was one of those coaches who should have believed my own eyes and not been sucked in by group-think. As Steven Levitt and Stephen Dubner said in *Think Like a Freak*, "The conventional wisdom is often wrong."

The older, somewhat-shaky evidence against the use of weighted sleds led us to undervalue and underutilize a valuable piece of equipment. To generate even more confusion, a few authors stated that the weighted sled didn't improve speed, but did indicate sled training would improve acceleration.

One major problem is that we may have misinterpreted the results of the early sled research. Most coaches spend too much time working on form running and technique in the attempt to improve speed. These same coaches also include lower-body strength workouts to improve strength.

Although these may both be important, there may be a few missing links. One I alluded to previously was the obvious act of running timed sprints. The other was the development of specific strength. All too often, we see athletes who run "pretty" but not fast. Many coaches attempting to develop speed spend far too much time on technique drills and far too little on developing the specific power and strength necessary to run faster.

In 2000, *The Journal of Applied Physiology* published an article called "Mechanical Basis of Human Running Speed." The article synopsis begins with the line, "Faster top running speeds are achieved with greater ground forces, not more rapid leg movements." This became known as "the Weyand Study," named after lead researcher Peter Weyand. In an interesting twist, Weyand has recently disagreed with his own earlier study, citing stride frequency as more important. More evidence that research

Chapter 11—Speed Development

changes and that science is really about questioning the science.

In any case, weighted sled drills target the specific muscles used in sprinting and should be viewed as a form of *horizontal strength and power training*. I now refer to sled sprints as "horizontal Olympic lifts." By this, I mean they're a horizontal power exercise we can train with purpose through the monitoring of speed and load.

The key here is the correct combination of speed *and* load. Cam Josse crunched the numbers and boiled the research on sled training for speed improvement down to this:

"Select a load that yields a sprint time that is 150% of your sprint time for the same distance."

Morin referred to this as a speed decrement.

For example, if your male athlete runs the 10 in 1.5 seconds, select a load that has him sled sprinting around 2.25 seconds for 10 yards. It's simple—just do the math.

Cam made it even simpler. He said, "Just aim for 2 to 2.3 seconds for 10 yards and you'll get the right load." Under 2 seconds? Add weight to the sled. Over 2.3, take some off.

In our case, we use our same fly-10 setup and aim for 150% of the fly 10. As our athletes cover 20 yards and we time the last 10, we use the fly-10 times with a 10-yard fly-in as the starting point. This means athletes who run under 1.2 must be under 1.7 or 1.8 and athletes who run 1.3 must be under 1.9. Currently our athletes are using anywhere from 65 to 135 pounds for these speed-and-distance combos, and we simply say "be under 2 seconds."

One big point of emphasis: Surface matters. The age of the turf, turf versus rubber and other variables will all influence sled times. Loads placed on the sled are different on grass than on turf and will even vary with rain or temperature changes. This simply relates to the coefficient of friction.

Pushing a heavy sled or sprinting with a weighted sled teaches strong athletes how to produce the type of force that moves them forward. Sports scientists often like to break this down into "special strength" and "specific strength." Although I believe the difference is minimal, it can help to understand the difference.

"Special strength" refers to movements with resistance that incorporate the joint dynamics of the skill. Sled marching falls into the special strength category. Sled marching may be one of the best tools we have for speed development. An athlete's inability to produce force in the action of sprinting becomes glaringly obvious in sled marching.

Loads far exceeding an athlete's body weight can be used for special strength work as long as the athlete exhibits a similar sprint motor pattern. This means sled marching should look like a sprint drill and not like pushing a car out of a snow bank. Think of the sled march as a closed-chain unilateral leg press.

Athletes incorporate the joint dynamics of sprinting through hip extension and hyperextension against resistance. This can be an extremely heavy movement as long as we get a technically sound marching action, meaning perfect posture. We aren't talking about sled dragging here, rather a sled march is a crisp marching action.

We've taken this idea a step further and now treat our sled march like any other strength exercise. Marches are now done for reps instead of distance. This means if the program calls for three sets of eight reps, we do three sets for eight reps (steps) each leg. Heavy pushes use the push sleds and for the lighter sprints, we use the flat towing sleds.

"Specific strength" is defined as movement with resistance that's imitative of the joint action. I place sled sprinting in the specific-strength category.

In the past, coaches suggested that resisted speed development work must not slow the athlete down more than 10% or must not involve more than 10% of the athlete's body weight. These recommendations were based on motor-learning research that indicated excessive loads would alter the motor patterns of activities like sprinting or throwing. I've always felt there was a missing link to speed development, but this so-called "10% rule" kept me from aggressively pursuing my gut feeling.

The beauty in sled sprinting is that loads that are too heavy *look too heavy*. When selecting loads based on speed change and not on a percentage of body weight, sled sprints look like sled sprints. When the load is too heavy, it's obvious.

With this method, we now see loads up to 75% of body weight, but that doesn't matter. It's not about the weight on the sled but about the time/speed decrement. This only really becomes a problem with larger athletes like football linemen. They already have strength-to-bodyweight issues;

using percentages of larger body weights vs speed decrement can really slow a large athlete down. A simpler rule? The heavier the athlete, the lighter the starting weight on the sled.

Another failing of the so-called 10% rule is that it doesn't allow us to apply progressive resistance concepts to this form of training.

All of our athletes do sled work; I think of the heavy sled pushes as a great posterior-chain exercise. Charlie Francis used a reverse leg press done on an old Universal Gym to emphasize the posterior chain. (see figure 7.29) The weighted sled is just a better version of this.

A sled may be the most underrated tool for speed development due to our misinterpretation and misunderstanding of the research and terminology surrounding speed development.

Planning Your Sled Workouts

Think of the sled pushing as a set of 10 reps, meaning steps. You want steps 9 and 10 to be somewhat difficult in the heavy pushing phase. Obviously, the type of sled, type of surface and other factors matter, but loads tend to be in excess of 2x body weight.

When I talk about a set of 10 reps, I'm referring to steps per leg. We're looking for a way to equalize everything. Using a set distance favors the taller athlete. But if we program 5 steps or 10 steps per leg, it's like doing a 5- or 10-rep set.

For sled sprints, the load is selected based on time. We want the sprint time to be 150% of the best time for 10 yards. Our athletes effectively sled sprint 20 yards, timing the last 10. For this, we're using up to 135 pounds for men and 45–90 for women.

Our first two phases (heavy sled pushes) are done as part of our strength work and fall into the category of specific strength. In phases three and four, we either run sled sprints after our sprints and plyos (before strength), or use them as part of a posterior-chain complex in a complex training phase.

While some coaches program contrast sprints by towing, releasing the sled and then sprinting, we don't due to logistics. I worry about people pushing or pulling sleds while others are sprinting. We'd need a larger area than we have and would need specially designed harnesses for this. We will, however, contrast a sled sprint with an unweighted sprint in later phases and have even done three part contrasts of sled push, sled sprint and sprint.

At times we have also done sled work four times per week. However, only two days are linear—the other two days are heavier crossover pushes or pulls. In the past few years, we've often had to eliminate the crossovers, again due to logistics.

I don't like using sled pushes for conditioning. The exception in my mind might be football linemen because that's what they do.

Conditioning with a loaded sled is hard, but relatively non-specific. When it comes time to condition, we tend to bike, run and slide board.

I dislike sled dragging (facing the sled) because of the prolonged lumbar flexion loads. In a general sense, it doesn't seem healthy. First responders might need small amounts of dragging for short distances, but very few first responders drag great distances.

I also don't like sled drags in adult fitness programs. Most adults spend their days in flexion and don't need more of it. Notice that we're talking about flexion loads—loads that pull with flexion forces.

To summarize, I love pushes, am okay with harnessed forward pulls, hate reverse drags and love crossovers. We do occasionally have our athletes perform reverse walks, particularly those with knee issues, but we have them use waist belts instead of handles.

Training Agility

Training agility is another interesting concept. I've never been a big fan of training agility as it tends to be lots of random running from cone to cone. In order to understand agility, we must decide what we think agility actually is, and once we do, we have to decide how it's best trained.

There are always coaches who post agility ladder videos and tell us what a waste of time the agility ladder is. In my mind, the agility ladder isn't a waste of time as long as you know why you're using it.

We love the ladder as a multi-planar warm-up tool. Agility ladders allow us to move in the frontal and transverse planes in warm-ups. And… athletes like agility ladders. Good warm-up, good engagement, good idea?

Many coaches continue to paint with a broad brush and color any pre-programmed agility drill as a bad idea. This is a classic example of turning a good idea into a bad idea.

In general, though, we don't do much agility work at MBSC. Most agility work is, in my mind, just running around. Coaches waste lots of time running people from cone to cone and then trying to get them to do it faster. That, to me, is a waste of time.

The big trend now is reactive agility. That's what occurs in a good practice and in things like small area games.

The whole "agility" idea grew out of American football not being a year-round sport. There may be a need to construct drills or scenarios to develop agility or direction-change skills in athletes who aren't able to play their sports year-round. Fortunately or unfortunately, for nearly everyone else—the non-American football athletes—there's generally a year-round aspect of skill development.

Too many coaches in sports other than American football are far too influenced by the training of these football players. If you work in a sport that can't be played in the off-season, there may be a need for agility work. However, most athletes are filling that bucket through practice and individual skill work.

At MBSC, we try to make agility development part of our warm-ups. We'll use an agility ladder for two or three minutes to move in multiple planes and to teach stabilization, landing and crossover skills. I also consider most of our single-leg work and single-leg plyos essential deceleration efforts that play a big part in agility development.

I think drills like 5–10–5 are kind of dumb. I can take 10 minutes and make people faster at it, but I don't think that will make them more agile. Then we get into the strength and eccentric strength parts. Does the athlete have the requisite strength to put on the brakes to cause a direction change?

Agility is a sequence of an eccentric contraction to a brief isometric to a concentric contraction. In order to be able to change direction, the athlete must be able to brake effectively. That braking action must then rapidly be converted back to another concentric contraction. I'm not sure that is teachable if athletes lack the requisite unilateral strength.

Athletes need exceptional single-leg strength or agility drills are a waste of time. I think our current widespread ACL problem is in large part due to this. Today's athletes generally have big engines and bad brakes, or in the case of female athletes, small engines and no brakes.

Sports like lacrosse, hockey and soccer can use simple three v two and two v one games to work on agility. In soccer, some teams swear by The Rondo, a soccer version of "keep away."

There are lots of opportunities in practice settings to fill the agility bucket.

Can We Improve Agility?

I can't tell you how often I hear a parent or coach ask, "How can I improve my kid's foot speed or agility?" Everyone wants a shortcut and a quick fix.

The better question might be, "Do you think we can improve foot speed?" Or maybe even the next question, "Does foot speed even matter?" That begs the larger question, "Does foot speed have anything to do with agility?"

I know coaches reading this are thinking, "What am I reading? Is this guy crazy?"

How many times have we heard that speed kills? The problem is that coaches and parents equate fast feet with moving fast and quick feet with being agile. However, having "fast feet" doesn't mean fast any more than having "quick feet" means agile. In some cases, fast feet might actually make athletes slow.

I often see fast feet as a detriment to speed. In fact, some of our quick turnover guys, those who'd be described as having fast feet, are very slow off the start. The problem with fast feet is that these athletes don't use the ground well to produce force. Fast feet might be good on hot coals, but not on hard ground.

Think of the ground as the well from which we draw speed. It's not how fast the feet move, but rather how much force goes into the ground. This is basic action-and-reaction physics.

Force into the ground equals forward or lateral motion. This is why athletes with the best vertical jumps are most often the fastest. It comes down to force production.

Often, coaches argue the "vertical versus horizontal" concept, claiming that a vertical jump doesn't correspond to horizontal speed. Years of data from the NFL Combine begs to differ. Force into the ground is force into the ground.

Coaches should be asking about vertical jump improvement, not about fast feet. My standard line is, "Michael Flatley has fast feet, but he doesn't really go anywhere. If you move your feet fast and don't go anywhere, does it matter?"

The best solution to slow feet is stronger legs. Feet don't matter. Legs matter.

If you stand at the starting line and take a quick first step but fail to push with the other leg, you don't go anywhere. The reality is that a quick first step is actually the result of a powerful first push. We should change the buzzwords and start to say, "That kid has a great first push."

Think about this for a minute: Feet can't be quick. They're simply the ground contacts stuck to the bottom of our legs. Blade Runner Oscar Pistorius was the finest example of this—he had no feet. Even if he wanted his feet to move faster, that action would primarily have to come from the hips. Imagine a coach saying, "He needs faster hips."

But that's not really our topic. I'm simply trying to redefine a bad term: first step, as in, "He has a great first step," or "She needs to work on her first step." A great first step is actually a powerful first push. To top it off, the power for that first step comes not from the stepping foot, but from the other foot. Confused? You shouldn't be.

If you want to get by someone in front of you and you step with your right foot, the power, speed and quickness are actually generated by the left foot.

We don't have a great first step as much as *having a powerful first push*. If we start to talk about it this way, maybe we can get people to stop doing all kinds of silly foot quickness drills and start working on strength and power.

Lower-body strength might be the real cure for slow feet and the real key to speed and to agility. The essence of developing quick feet lies in single-leg strength and single-leg stability work—landing skills. If you can't decelerate, you can't accelerate, at least not more than once.

I love the idea of a magic drill. This is the theory that developing foot speed and agility isn't a process of gaining strength and power, but rather the lack of a specific drill. If I believed there was a magic drill, we'd do it every day. But in fact, it comes down to horsepower and the nervous system, two areas that change slowly over time.

In spite of the negativity around ladders, I love ladder drills. They provide an excellent multi-planar dynamic warm-up. They develop a brain-to-muscle connection and are excellent for eccentric strength and stability. We do less than five minutes of ladder drills one or two times a week. I don't believe for a minute that the ladder is a magic tool that will make our athletes faster or more agile; however,

I do believe it's a piece of the puzzle from the neural perspective.

People waste more than five minutes on biceps curls, but we have long debates about doing ladder drills. Ladder drills are also a great tool to put on a show for coaches who want foot speed work. Sometimes it's easier to give a "yes" than to argue with them.

What I don't love is the jump rope, particularly as an agility tool. Give a guy with "bad feet" a jump rope, and you get a guy with bad feet and patellar tendonitis.

Also, we never use the term "speed ladder." We always call it an "agility ladder" if we call it anything other than a ladder.

So, how do we develop speed, quickness and agility? Unfortunately, we need to do it the slow, old-fashioned way. You can play with ladders and bungee cords all you want, but that's like putting mag wheels on an Escort. The real key is to increase the horsepower, the brakes and the accelerator.

Development of speed, agility and quickness simply comes down to good training. We need to work on lower-body strength and lower-body power, and we need to do it on one leg.

Plyometric Updates

We've made very few changes in our plyo programs in the past 20 years. I know that sounds crazy, but we've followed the same simple program all these years.

In 2019, we switched our medial/lateral hops from a straight frontal-plane movement to a 45-degree angle with a forward translation. This was simply because most decelerative foot contacts are much closer to 45 degrees than 90. This was a small point, but was a large change for us.

A second change was eliminating the gravity-reduced component of phase one. We've always jumped "up" to a box in our linear phase-one jumps and hops.

However, in the interest of getting to true reactive plyometrics sooner, we found ourselves starting in what many would recognize as phase two, jumping and hopping over obstacles.

Chapter 11—Speed Development

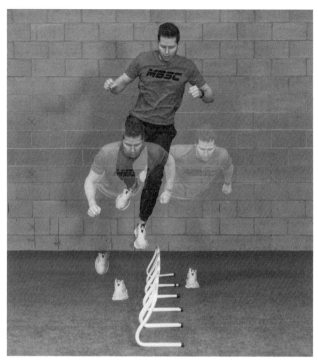

Figure 11.1—Medial or lateral hops, the first big change to our plyometric program in decades.

There were two thoughts here. Many of our programs have been running 9 or 10 weeks versus 12. This means we'd be using three phases instead of four. For us, reactive plyos are our last phase, and in our former progression, we often never got to the true "react, resist, repel" stages of jumps and hops.

This meant we were forced to make a change, and that change was to eliminate some of our phase-one box jumps and box hops.

Hopping same foot to same foot is theoretically less difficult, but in actuality is more difficult and riskier, which is a big issue. A single-leg box hop (hopping up) is psychologically a greater challenge than a single-leg hurdle hop (hopping over).

The inclusion of more power skips was another change we made. We've never had success with forward bounds and simply avoided them. However, we found that from a speed standpoint, we needed a unilateral plyometric that focused on horizontal translation. Power skips are perfect for this.

The Mini-Bounce Phase

If you've followed our MBSC methods, you'll know our plyo progression moves from "sticking the landing" in phase one to adding a mini-bounce in phase two. The truth is, our phase one plyos aren't really plyometrics drills, but rather are jumping and landing drills. Our initial emphasis is on landing mechanics and developing tendon strength.

In phase two, we add a mini-bounce. Here, rather than trying to react powerfully to the ground, we create a transition phase where we try to get the athletes to feel a bounce.

I've always believed this was a valuable phase, but lacked a scientific explanation. Listening to Australian physical therapist Jill Cook (Jake Turra's Jacked Athlete podcast) gave me the scientific explanation for something we'd done intuitively for decades. We followed the progression the way we did to avoid patella-femoral irritation—sore knees from jumping.

We knew if we took our time and progressed from sticking to mini-bounces and eventually to "real" plyos, we'd get to our destination with healthy knees. We just didn't know why.

Cook pointed out that the highest tendon stress was at the point of switching from an eccentric contraction to a concentric contraction. Adding a phase that eases into that eccentric-to-concentric switch adds another layer of tendon preparation. It's a layer that seems to help injury-proof our athletes.

Depth Jumps?

A recent X/Twitter video brought depth drops back into the picture. The athlete in the online video "drops" off a stacked pile of plyo boxes about two meters in height, and then goes into a rebound jump. Some coaches marveled at the athleticism. I cringed at the stupidity and what that stupidity might lead to.

And then I let my feelings be known. This, of course, led to a number of "why not?" responses from some coaches. The worst part for me was being written off by some as a social media "influencer."

First off, let's attempt to define what was shown in the video. Technically, the video was a depth drop to a rebound. The athlete didn't attempt to re-jump, but instead seemed to simply react elastically to the ground. Imagine dropping a basketball from six feet.

Yuri Verkhoshansky advocated what he called "depth jumps" and recommended a height of three-quarters of a meter to one meter (30 to 40 inches). Pavo Komi—and later Carmelo Bosco—advocated a drop jump from 60 centimeters (24 inches). Although similar, they had some differences. Bosco also felt that heights higher than 60 centimeters could be dangerous.

In the cases of both Verkhoshansky and Bosco, the goal was to use the force of gravity to overload the muscle-tendon unit.

The net result of these so-called "shock methods" was in some cases elite performance, and in other cases it was injury. These types of exercises were popular in the late 1970s and early '80s.

"The way drop jumping has become popular is typical of how training methods evolve. It is rumored that the Russian athlete who won the 100 and 200m dash in the 1972 Olympics, Valery Borzov, utilized plyometric drills as part of his training (Wilt, 1978). Coaches of rival athletes became interested and began to search for more information. They found a description of drop jumping in a translated Russian paper by Verkhoshansky (1966), and adopted the idea and developed their own modifications. These modifications are now incorporated in widespread athletic programs."

Incredibly, in the late 1970s and early '80s, this led some coaches to take athletes out to jump off the back of bleachers. In our more-is-better world, we tossed caution to the wind and endangered lots of athletes. Because of the misuse and misunderstanding of this technique, we didn't advocate or use depth drops or depth jumps in our training.

However, in the last two years, we've experimented with some eccentric overload drops with no rebound. Our last change was the addition of depth drops in phase 1. I have been strongly anti-depth drop in the past because the exercise tended to be overdone to the point of being dangerous. However, the work of Coach Hunter Eisenhower and his study of the forces generated by depth drops forced us to reconsider and modify our position. It is important to note that depth drops (no rebound/re-jump) should start from only 10% higher than the athlete's best vertical jump in order to allow athletes to adapt to the forces created.

The athlete in the X/Twitter clip who started this discussion was dropping from greater than two meters. This could be in the neighborhood of 80–100% overload, assuming a vertical jump between 30 and 40 inches.

The X/Twitter rationale used to defend this extreme drop was that kids in play situations routinely jump down from heights that might approach their measured heights and that as result, depth jumps or drops are safe. This is a short-sighted rationale on a number of fronts.

In the simplest sense, we have to look at the idea that because a kid does it, it's therefore safe for adults and athletes.

Children are probably much more elastic than adults and also have far less mileage. Kids do lots of dumb things and survive, but that doesn't put those activities on a recommended list.

Although kids may jump down, we must ask about the frequency and volume of these landings. My guess is they're actually quite rare. In training athletes, I assume we'd do these types of drop landings regularly.

Kids may have "juicy tendons," but two of the leading childhood pain syndromes are Osgood-Schlatter disease (an overuse syndrome of the tibial tuberosity) and Sever's disease (an overuse syndrome of the Achilles insertion). Neither of these are actual diseases; they're overuse syndromes. My point here is that kids can and do get overuse syndromes similar to adults, and these issues may be caused by reckless play.

In sports, athletes never have to come down from higher than they can jump up. Production of these forces can only be artificially obtained. In the video that prompted these thoughts, the athlete actually uses a ladder to get to the top of the boxes.

My fear is that a video like this will fuel imitators. If experience teaches us anything, it's that people love to imitate cool stuff they see on the internet. I can see a depth drop craze similar to the high-box jump craze, with people attempting to survive higher and higher drops. Failure will be catastrophic as we wait for the inevitable gym fail video of a patellar tendon rupture.

Watching the video brought me back to the previously mentioned Jacked Athlete podcast where host Jake Tuura interviewed Jill Cook, one of the world's preeminent authorities on patellar tendon and patella-femoral issues. Cook thinks that depth drops are a really dumb idea. I can justify 10% higher than the best vertical jump in order to create on overload, but not nearly 100% more.

I messaged a young coach who praised the video and reminded him that when people seek to be social media influencers or content curators, it comes with a responsibility. We must exercise good judgment and caution, knowing that impressionable athletes and coaches are watching, listening and reading.

CHAPTER 12
CONDITIONING

My thoughts on conditioning have changed drastically over the last three decades. Thirty years ago, I thought that harder was better.

I was a classic old-school coach. We ran lots of tracks intervals—440s, 220s, 110s. The truth is, I was probably as dumb as a conditioning coach as I was as a strength coach. The only good thing was that we were still smarter than most and at least embraced interval training over the foolish distance running that was prevalent at the time.

Coaches are now saying that something like a 300-yard shuttle run is a bad conditioning test because it isn't specific to many sports. However, to frame the argument, it's important to give you some historical perspective. In the early 1990s, I had to fight our football coach to get him to stop making our entire team do a 1.5-mile Cooper test. Imagine offensive linemen training to get to a mile-and-a-half in under 12 minutes. It was bad.

Almost everyone was some kind of dumb. Along the same lines, hockey players were doing VO_2 max tests to determine "fitness." Basketball players and soccer players were also regularly being tested at distances like one-and-a-half to two miles. Trust me, tests like 16 x 110 or the 300 shuttle were major improvements in the conditioning process.

Over the years, we at MBSC have done less and less conditioning. Most of our athletes, both high school and professional, are now playing their sports year-round for multiple hours a week.

In fact, it's not unusual for our athletes to do no conditioning with us. Our current policy is that if you have a practice or skill session, you don't need to condition that day.

Killing the Goose That Lays the Golden Eggs

Years ago, I heard Dan Pfaff tell a story. It's a wonderful tale of intelligence and humility.

"In the early 1970s, I was a high school coach in rural SW Ohio. We were a small school, and athletes often played whatever sport was in season. Our basketball team was a district power, small but tenacious. They full-court pressed the entire game, *so these guys could run for days. Two of the most enduring players caught my eye as I recruited for the upcoming track season, and I approached the guys about coming out to run. They were hesitant, but the head coach gave his blessing, stating that it was a good way to stay in shape. Travel teams and AAU basketball hadn't been invented yet, so guys just played pickup ball in the off-season, and the coach was worried about their conditioning over the long off-season.*

Our basketball season ended in early March with the state playoffs. Track season began at the end of March, so I gave the guys a few weeks off, and we started training them later that month. I didn't enter them in the first meet as we had to figure out which events they were best suited for and to assess fitness for those events. I did extensive varieties of running sessions and the data said these guys would best fit as 400m/800m types, so that's the way we went.

After a few weeks of training, we entered a low-key dual meet, and both guys broke the existing school record. The next weekend, they broke it again, and I was strutting around like a genius coach. Their times projected them to be state qualifiers, so I really hit the books finding key training ideas and sessions.

By the end of the season, neither guy even made the district meet. I'd coached both of them to slower times with my magic sessions. Two-second drop-off from early season results…that's when I had the "ah ha" awakening that basketball activities did a pretty good job of training components necessary for these events in track, and that my bias had derailed the train. Lesson learned. The next year, they played ball three days a week and did just one or two designed sessions on the track… both were district finalists."

The moral of the story? Don't outsmart yourself. Don't kill the goose that lays the golden eggs.

It's significantly easier to get an explosive athlete "in shape" than it is to make an "in shape" athlete explosive. The first will take weeks, the second may take years. Think about that every time you design a conditioning program.

Sport-Specific Conditioning?

As you may already know, I hate the term "sport-specific training" and rarely use it. However, when it comes to conditioning, training should be as sport-specific as possible. At a bare minimum, conditioning should at least be specific to groups of sports. When developing sport-specific conditioning programs, the key is to look at the field, the substitution patterns and the energetics of the game. It's not how far athletes run in a game, but at what pace and over what time period.

Distance running advocates often default to the mileage covered in a game as rationalization for long slow distance conditioning. However, as they like to say in the NFL, upon further review things change a bit. In a game like soccer, a player can easily cover five kilometers in a game; however, the majority of the distance covered is actually walked, not jogged or sprinted. In conditioning, specifics matter.

The process of strength training and conditioning for many sports has progressed from a Stone Age approach of utilizing training camp to get in shape to a more modern approach based on the utilization of in-season and off-season training programs. We now have GPS units and heart rate monitors to quantify lots of what "we thought."

Unfortunately, conditioning and conditioning testing continue to be controversial. Some coaches are bringing back the long slow stuff and touting "Zone 2 work." Other coaches see conditioning tests as a game of "Can You Top This." If your team does two 300 shuttles for testing, another team will out-work you and do three. If your team runs 16 110s, another team will run 32. Conditioning testing has moved from an evaluation of preparedness to a contest of excesses.

Conditioning isn't meant for mental toughness; it's meant to create preparedness for practice and game situations. If we're injuring our players or making them slower in the conditioning process, we aren't enhancing performance—we're detracting from it.

While this chapter isn't intended to provide a physiology lesson, it'll hopefully prompt some coaches to consider the application of more specific concepts to their sports.

Evaluating Conditioning

Some groups still adhere to the idea that all athletes need to develop an aerobic base. I'm not sure why people felt so compelled to develop an aerobic base, and more importantly, why we thought we needed to develop this base through long slow training. No one has adequately explained this need for an aerobic base. I think it's simply an assumption that things will work better if we have that base.

Luckily, we seem to have moved away from the idea that the overall fitness of an athlete is based on maximum oxygen consumption (Max VO_2). MVO_2 is a standard measure of aerobic capacity originally intended to evaluate the conditioning of athletes involved in endurance sports.

In the 1980s and 1990s, the influence of exercise physiologists was heavily felt, and misinformation tended to trickle down to all levels of sports. Asking physiologists to evaluate fitness or conditioning for team sports may have been a case of the old "when the only tool you have is a hammer, everything looks like a nail." Exercise physiologists don't necessarily have a ton of tools in the toolbox, so they tended to go to the tools they had.

We didn't have a standard test for each sport that could be mutually agreed upon by both exercise scientists and members of the coaching community, and that was a problem. Thankfully, many sports have progressed from the old "Cooper Test 12-Minute Run" philosophy to the use of tests like the 300-yard shuttle or the yo-yo intermittent recovery tests (beep tests).

Using Performance Tests

Based on my experience, I believe there's at least one fatal flaw in using physiological data to evaluate performance of athletes. Physiological data like MVO_2 or lactate threshold are measures of physiological variables, not performance variables. Physiological testing may tell us something about the inner workings of an athlete, but the information obtained is suspect at best.

Energy systems authority Paul Robbins of EXOS often refers to MVO_2 as a measure of what someone "might" do. Why might? In sports conditioning and in the testing of conditioning, success is as much mental as it is physical. The most aerobically fit athletes, when measured by VO_2 often don't get the highest scores on performance tests. Whether we use the yo-yo test, the 300-yard shuttle run, a two-mile run or a two-mile Assault Bike session, we don't tend to see any correlation to physiological tests.

I believe all testing should be performance-based for athletes because we want to see what they're capable of in head-to-head competition. I don't care if one athlete can use more oxygen or accumulate less lactate than another. I want to see who will come in first when I line them up and test them.

Athletes find physiological testing both frustrating and confusing because it tends to reward physiology over performance. Instead, evaluative testing should be performance-based. If you're going to evaluate athletes, give them a chance to do what they do best: compete.

In the physiological testing of our 2004 Boston University hockey players, the athlete who lasted the longest on our treadmill test only scored a 52 on our VO_2 test. How do I tell an athlete he's in poor shape when he watched the test and knows he ran twice as long as the guy who was in "better shape"?

Personally, I'll leave fitness evaluation to competitive testing in which the success or failure is obvious. The person who comes in first is in the best shape.

Target heart rate is another flawed physiological assumption. For my 18- to 22-year-old collegians, the theoretical target heart rate would be a max of 198–202. Our range when actually tested was 180–211. When we do heart-rate–dictated training, the assumption of 220 minus age would result in overtraining for some and undertraining for others. The idea of 220 minus age is valid to within one standard deviation for 70% of the population. The other 30% can be as much as two standard deviations from the theoretical norm. This could be a variance of up to 22 beats per minute.

If you want to do heart-rate–based training, the best bet is to do some type of max effort test—we use a two-mile Assault Bike ride—and assume the highest heart rate attained during the test to be 95–100%.

Are Most Sports Aerobic Sports?

This is the million-dollar question. And of course, the answer is no. But if most sports aren't aerobic sports, why do we still have teams emphasizing aerobic capacity?

Teams often emphasize aerobic capacity for their players because of the belief that an efficient aerobic system promotes faster recovery. Yet, this philosophy may lead to the creation of slower athletes who can rapidly recover to attempt to regain all the ground they lost to the faster athletes.

Another reason many teams emphasize aerobic training is that it's easy to perform and implement, particularly when compared to training for speed and power. It's much easier to demand volume and effort than for coaches to learn the finer points of speed and power development.

However, the questions really begin at this point. An efficient aerobic system will facilitate faster recovery. But are we enhancing the recovery ability of an athlete we've made slower? At what cost are we developing the aerobic system, and how do we do it?

Physiological principles tell us that muscle fibers respond to training. Are we training explosive anaerobic athletes and in our zeal to enhance their recovery ability, making them slower? In truth, most team sports have a highly anaerobic component that puts a tremendous stress on the adenosine triphosphate, phosphate creatine (ATP-PC) and lactic acid (LA) systems.

During most games, players perform a series of three- to five-second sprints. Very rarely is a player actually running at a steady-state pace for any length of time.

It would appear the aerobic demand of that sequence would be fairly low. However, the demands on the athletes' speed, speed endurance and acceleration is high.

My theory (based on Charlie Francis's early work) proposes that for many players, particularly young developing players, any emphasis on aerobic conditioning through steady-state exercise might actually be counterproductive.

Are Aerobic Adaptations Desirable?

One of the major drawbacks of aerobic training is that it *may* compromise speed at the cellular level. Some of the adaptations of muscle to aerobic training are in direct opposition to the primary needs of most athletes.

In Charlie Francis's book *Training for Speed,* he makes a number of thought-provoking points regarding the training of the sprinter. And…aren't all team sport athletes sprinters?

Quoting *Training for Speed:*

"Enough power-related work must be done during the early years (ages 13 to 17) to:

- *Maintain genetically determined levels of white or power-related muscle fiber.*
- *And promote the shift of transitional or intermediate fiber to white power-related muscle fiber."*

Francis further stated, "Endurance work must be carefully limited to light or light/medium volumes to prevent the conversion of transitional or intermediate muscle fiber to red endurance muscle fiber."

This may be one of the most important statements about the training of an athlete you'll ever read. I can state with conviction that these concepts have formed the essence of my thought processes for the last 35 years and may be the key to the long-term development of athletes both young and old.

I always joke that I know the key to making a kid lousy at sports: early endurance training. If you want a child to be slow, start endurance training as soon as you finish reading this. In the 1990s, I watched older players train themselves out of their leagues or sports by adhering to the aerobically oriented off-season programs of their teams.

A quick reminder: A highly skilled player may not be as adversely affected as a marginal one. Marginal players at most levels generally have lower vertical jumps and anaerobic power than their more highly skilled counterparts. These players are already at a disadvantage that'll only be magnified by an aerobically oriented training program.

Muscles are made up of three types of fibers: fast twitch (anaerobic), slow twitch (aerobic) and intermediate. The ratio of fast-twitch fibers to slow-twitch fibers is one of the primary determinants of success in team sports. The best way to estimate fast-twitch capability is through vertical jump testing and 10-yard dash testing.

Charlie Francis noted that, "Young athletes who do not achieve high levels of oxygen uptake during a treadmill test but who perform well over 10- to 40-meter sprints probably have inherited a high proportion of white power-related muscle fibers."

Current theory leads coaches to assume that athletes with low MVO_2 values are out of shape. In fact, these athletes probably possess the exact quantity those coaches are looking for. At Boston University, many of our talented hockey players who went on to long NHL careers were the worst performers in tests that evaluate aerobic capacity.

An athlete with a high vertical jump and poor aerobic capacity will be a better prospect for team sports than one with great aerobic capacity and poor explosive power. Athletes with predominantly fast-twitch fibers will excel in sprint-oriented sports such as soccer or hockey, but will struggle in aerobic activities. Those with predominantly slow-twitch fibers will excel at endurance-oriented sports. Most educated readers shouldn't be surprised at this.

However, what happens to the intermediate fibers is most likely a result of the training program. A program emphasizing long aerobic workouts will cause the intermediate fibers to adapt the characteristics of slow-twitch fibers. One emphasizing interval sprints with longer recovery will promote the movement of intermediate fibers toward the anaerobic, fast-twitch fibers.

Anaerobics to Develop the Aerobic System?

Conventional aerobic training (long slow distance) should be done only as frequently as is absolutely necessary—and that might be never. Instead, the aerobic system should be developed as a byproduct of anaerobic training. Interval training—anaerobic intervals—will generally keep the recovery heart rate in the aerobic range (over 120 BPM) if the intervals are done intensely enough.

This type of training will develop aerobic capacity, but as a byproduct of the anaerobic work. This is obviously a more sport-specific method of training the aerobic capabilities of an anaerobic athlete.

Sport-Specific Testing

A player's conditioning level should be determined by a battery of tests that relate to the sport, not by a MVO_2 test or a timed distance run. MVO_2 tells a coach that a player has an efficient aerobic system. So what? A player's conditioning level should be based on a number of tests.

Another trendy idea is to check blood lactate values. Again, this is a physiological measurement and not a performance measurement. Athletes become frustrated when they perform well on performance testing and are then told they are "out of shape" based on a physiologist's analysis of data.

Specific conditioning tests need to be developed to test conditioning relative to each sport's demand.

Soccer

For soccer, the yo-yo intermittent recovery test—commonly referred to as the "beep test"—has great value. This test is also applicable to sports like field hockey, lacrosse and to a lesser degree, basketball. It's a beautifully simple test of fitness and willpower. Athletes compete until failure.

I've seen soccer coaches praise an athlete in one breath for a strong beep test performance, and then a day later declare the person unfit based on physiological data. This is foolish. Believe what you see; believe in performance. I can't overstate the fact that physiological testing doesn't transfer into performance. Performance is as much about heart and will as it is about physiology.

Ice Hockey

Ice hockey players will benefit more from a test like the 300-yard shuttle run. The 300-yard shuttle run consists of two 300-yard runs done on either a 25-yard (12 x 25) or a 50-yard (6 x 50) course done with five minutes rest between runs. Due to the truly intermittent nature of ice hockey, a test of repeated efforts with a recovery period in between is a better indicator of actual fitness for hockey than any other available test.

We've developed an on-ice version of the 300 shuttle. The test consists of two bouts of seven trips from the near blue line to the goal line. This test closely mimics the 300 shuttle but is done on ice.

Football

Football players benefit more from a series of seven-second runs followed by a slightly longer recovery. Years ago, we modified the 16 110-yard run test first popularized by Miami Heat strength coach Bill Foran into a 24 x 55-yard test more specific to the energy demands of football. The original 16 110-yard sprint test was developed in the 1980s and consisted of 110-yard sprints, followed by an approximately 40- to 45-second recovery period. Players were required to make times based on position group. Linemen ran somewhere in the 18-second range, while skill- position players were required to run in the 15- to 16-second range.

In the modified version, the original thought was to cut the distance in half and double the number of repetitions. I found this (32 x 55) was overly ambitious and settled on 24 x 55-yard run at a slightly faster pace. Linemen were given nine seconds; linebackers, tight ends and fullbacks were given eight seconds; and skill-position players had 7.5 seconds. This is a difficult test due to all of the acceleration and deceleration.

There's conflict and confusion around football conditioning testing. I think over time we may develop even better methods to test fitness for American football, but a repeat run ability isn't a bad place to start.

Recap of Testing

The key to testing is to look at the demands of each sport and not to simply do what everyone else is doing. Try to envision what would be the best test for your athletes at their level. If you're working with young athletes, be even more careful.

Here's the big problem with testing of any type: *Athletes will train for the test.* If you want your athletes to train for speed and power but you test for aerobic capacity, you can rest assured your athletes will be training for aerobic capacity.

What Makes a Successful Player?

If you doubt what I'm saying, ask yourself what makes a successful player in the sport. Success in most sports is highly dependent on skill. However, if the quality of skill is assumed, the next most valuable quality in team sports would be speed.

The training program should resemble that of a sprinter. The emphasis should be on developing the power of the legs and hips through lower-body weight training, plyometrics and sprinting.

For most sports, the majority of conditioning should be interval training done on a field, a slide board or, for athletes with injury problems, a bike.

Conditioning program effectiveness is drastically increased when using a heart rate monitor. Don't bother with the expensive models. For our hockey players, we've gone to a system of self-paced interval training based on individual heart-rate response. The athletes are told:

How many intervals to perform

How many beats of recovery heart rate to use

Strength and Conditioning Coaching

For most athletes, we recommend a 40-beat-per-minute recovery. For athletes who routinely top 170, we recommend a 50-beat-per-minute recovery period. Each athlete recovers at his or her own ability based on the reaction of the heart to training. Some athletes may perform the majority of a workout at a one-to-one rest-to-work ratio, while others will be two to one or even three to one.

Each athlete performs a self-paced workout but can't cheat due to the presence of the heart rate monitor. This ensures that we won't overtrain unfit athletes or undertrain fit athletes. With the price of heart rate monitors so low, I believe this type of training will become much more common.

Think about an old-fashioned interval workout. Everyone would be told the distance to run, the time to run that distance and the rest time. This is incredibly arbitrary. The assumption is that the time of the work interval is all that matters. But instead of good training, more fit athletes may be having an easy day, while the less fit athlete is actually working too hard. Basing a workout on actual recovery versus an arbitrary ratio of rest to work is logical.

Interval Training and Knee Pain

Many athletes avoid running due to knee problems—or fear of them. However, most knee pain is caused by distance running, not interval training. Interval training is usually tougher on the muscles and the mind than on the joints. I rarely see athletes who can't interval train due to knee pain, but the repeated foot strikes of jogging are problematic. Athletes with patella-femoral pain (or any other lower-body overuse problem) are encouraged to ride a stationary bike.

Time Expectations
for Change of Direction Conditioning

The areas of conditioning that now need to be emphasized are muscular and movement specificity. Not enough programs address changes of direction as a vital component of sport conditioning. Most of the programs detailed in this chapter address change of direction as a key component of conditioning.

The ability to tolerate the muscular forces generated by accelerating and decelerating, and the ability to adapt to the additional metabolic stress caused by acceleration and deceleration,

are the real keys to conditioning. Deficiencies in these components are often why athletes describe themselves as "not being in game shape."

Many athletes train by running, or worse, riding a set distance in a set amount of time with no thought to the additional stresses provided by having to speed up and slow down. These are old-fashioned conditioning programs that operate on the oversimplified assumption that 30 seconds of exercise is always the same.

Ask athletes to perform a linear interval like a 220-yard run and then ask them to run a 150-yard shuttle run on a 25-yard course. Next, ask them to compare the feeling. Most athletes will describe the shuttle run as being much more difficult, yet both will be in the 30 second range.

Athletes are frequently injured in training camp settings in spite of following a prescribed conditioning program to the letter. This is usually due to following a conditioning program that ignores the three vital components of the conditioning process:

> *Acceleration*
> *Deceleration*
> *Change of direction*

Programs that force athletes to increase speed, decrease speed and change direction drastically reduce the incidence of early-season groin and hamstring injuries and better prepare them for the demands of an actual game or event.

Time Expectation Guidelines

The following time expectations are provided for information and comparison purposes. These times are estimates for Division I college athletes, professionals or Olympians. Please use them only as guidelines.

Shuttle Runs, 50- or 25-Yard Course

300-yard shuttle runs—55 seconds for a 50-yard course and 57–58 seconds for a 25-yard course (men) to 60 seconds for a 50-yard course and 62 seconds for a 25-yard course (women), followed by a 2- to 3-minute rest or a 40–50 beat recovery

150-yard shuttle runs—25–26 seconds for men and 28–30 seconds for women, followed by a 90-second rest

We avoid conventional long slow distance aerobic training. We don't spend any time focusing on an aerobic base or doing what's popularly referred to as "Zone 2 conditioning."

One final thought when developing conditioning programs: Don't increase the total time or total distance covered by more than 20% from week to week. A 20% increase will keep your athletes continuing to improve conditioning without an increased risk of injury. To monitor this, we calculate both total distance and total time.

Example: 5 x 150-yard shuttle run = 750 yards

The total time is approximately 2:30 of actual work based on an estimate of 30 seconds per 150-yard shuttle.

To stay within the 20% rule, the distance can't increase by more than 150 yards and the time by 30 seconds. You could either add an additional 150-yard shuttle or perform 1 x 300 yards and 4 x 150 yards. This would give you a total time of three minutes and a total distance of 900 yards. This is the key to injury prevention when designing conditioning programs.

Conditioning on the Assault AirBike

I've become a huge fan of bike conditioning, particularly when dealing with athletes who have multiple weekly sport practices. With multiple practices—and the often-simultaneous two-sport participation for high school kids—conditioning emphasis shifts to avoidance of muscle strains and overuse injury. At this point, additional work may best be done on a stationary bike if the athletes are also training on the field, ice or court.

Our old rationale for not using a bike—or any incomplete hip-extension apparatus—is the hip extensors and flexors not being properly prepared for the rigors of exercises like running or skating when athletes train on a bike.

Years ago, we actually had athletes who trained exclusively on a bike, Stairmaster or elliptical trainer in the off-season. The end result was often athletes with the energy system capability to finish a practice, but not the muscular ability. The athletes who didn't run on a regular basis didn't properly develop the hip flexors or extensors and were prone to hamstring and groin pulls.

Most aerobic exercise apparatus don't require or even allow for hip extension past neutral. On the opposite side, most of the recovery of the swing leg is passive. The result of off-season training centered on a piece of exercise equipment instead of running was often groin or hamstring strain in the preseason. The muscles simple aren't properly prepared for the stresses placed on it.

In the last 20 years, things have changed drastically. Instead of avoiding running off-season, we have nearly year-round running or skating.

In our current environment of nearly year-round sport participation, additional conditioning may be best done on a dual-action bike like the Assault.

Advantages of Dual-Action Bikes

Dual-action bikes mimic the combined arm-and-leg action of running or skating. A conventional bike uses only the legs.

The combination of arm-and-leg action produces a higher heart rate than pedaling alone. Arm action tends to elevate the heart rate approximately 10 BPM higher. This means the effect on the cardiovascular system is far more comparable to running or skating.

Dual-action fan-based bikes provide directly accommodating resistance. This is another often-overlooked benefit of a dual-action bike. The fan system delivers an equal and opposite reaction to the effort of the rider. There's no need to tighten a screw or to adjust the workload of the bike. The bike simply responds with greater air resistance to the effort of the rider.

Time and distance: Dual-action bikes tell the riders not only how long they've ridden, but also how far. This provides plenty of competitive opportunities.

Just a quick note: Hockey off-season conditioning has changed drastically in the past 10 years. When I originally wrote this book, players didn't skate in the summer (with the exception being a Thursday night beer league game), and teams actively encouraged extensive stationary bike work to raise MVO_2 levels.

Fast-forward 15 years and most players begin a formal skating program in early July. The result for us has been less running and more bike work

Strength and Conditioning Coaching

as the groin and hip-flexor area gets plenty of work through the on-ice sessions.

In much the same way, youth sports have also changed. Conditioning used to be a big priority. Kids needed to use the off-season to prepare for the season. Now, it seems like the seasons not only never end, but they even overlap. Kids are running or skating multiple times per week, and overuse is therefore the big enemy.

Several years ago, we switched from the Schwinn Airdyne to the Assault Bike. The Assault is basically a redesigned Airdyne, with the areas that tended to break down most frequently beefed up. Maintenance, the biggest issue with an Airdyne, is drastically reduced with an Assault.

I've always been a fan of these fan bikes (pun intended) because they allow work in a directly accommodating resistance format. Pedal harder, the task gets harder. It can't get simpler. No knobs to turn or buttons to push—just push the pedals.

Although I love for my hockey athletes to run in the off-season, we've had to curtail their running because the majority of our players now skate nearly year-round. When the season ends, there's a short time off, and then power skating begins. A large number of our players do some sort of skating program in conjunction with our summer strength and conditioning program. Stationary bike work allows us to get energy-system work without additional groin stress, and that means athletes stay healthier.

For our hockey athletes and our adult clients, the Assault allows us to get great energy-system work without the forward lean and resultant muscle shortening of a spin-type bike, and without the overuse injuries that are so much a part of jogging. In addition, the arm-and-leg dual action of the bike elevates the heart rate higher than a conventional bike.

The major problem we encountered when switching from the Schwinn to the Assault was in getting our athletes to understand the new numbers and times. Everyone was familiar with the Airdyne and had an idea of their times for certain distances and their workloads for intervals.

Unfortunately, as the Airdyne went through "improvements," we had different-sized fans, both big and small, and different computers. Although you might think this wouldn't matter, it did.

The easiest way to figure out a bike is to ride a mile at 60 RPMs and check the time. You can generalize this section to any of the dual-action bikes. However, the times are pretty specific. A mile at 60 RPMs takes 2:40 seconds on an Assault. All the times you read here are based on that.

A mile on the Airdyne, depending on model, took 2:30–2:45. A mile on the first-generation Assault was more in the 3:30–4:00 range. The new Assault—actually just a recalibrated head—is close to our old big-fan Airdyne times.

Now that we have them, how do we use the Assault bikes?

First, we get an MAS estimate. MAS is the acronym for maximum aerobic speed, basically the speed an athlete can maintain for about six minutes. We use a two-mile ride on the Assault bike. This generally takes between four-and-a-half and six minutes. From this two-mile test, we get an average RPM. The average RPM for two miles corresponds to the athlete's max aerobic speed (MAS). Here, max aerobic speed and average RPMs are synonymous.

We then program intervals at 110 or 120% of the MAS. I love the 20/10 and 10/20 built-in programs on the Assault for these types of intervals. We do 20/10 at 110% of MAS and 10/20 at 120%.

To provide numbers, if an athlete averaged 60 RPM for the 1.5-mile test (about 5:20), you'd program 20/10s trying to hit 66 RPMs (110% of 60) or better on each interval, and for 10/20, shoot for 72 RPM's (120% of 60). I got these MAS training percentages from Coach Dan Baker.

We do .2- and .3-mile repeats for our hockey players (50–60 seconds), again at 110–120% of MAS.

TIME EXPECTATIONS FOR WELL-CONDITIONED ATHLETES	
ASSAULT	
1 mi	2:30
3 mi	>8:00
5 mi	>13:40

Assault AirBike Elite?

We have about 20 Assaults and two of the Assault Elites. I have to admit I like the feel of the Elite better.

There are two issues.

The Elite costs about $400 dollars more than the Assault. That's a big deal in a commercial facility.

The computers are different. Although both bikes have a built-in 20/10 and 10/20 feature, the Elite doesn't log mileage during the rest periods. This may not seem like a big deal, but for us, we track total distance during a 20/10 or 10/20.

With the Original Assault, I generally log:

1.4 miles in a 20/10 set

1.2 miles in a 10/20

On the Elite, I only get 1.1 miles for a 20/10 because the bike only records the work portion of the ride. On the 10/20, I was only at .5 mile.

This is only a big deal if you're like me—meaning a bit OCD. I like to log the results of my rides. I've done over 900 rides and have times recorded since 2005 in a file in my computer. I like having the numbers.

12 Great Assault Bike Workouts

The following are 12 of our favorite workouts on the Assault.

Workout 1: Maximum Aerobic Speed Test

This is a two-mile time trial. Make this the first workout you use, as all others will be based on this.

In a perfect world, you'll get a two-mile time, an average RPM number, a one-minute recovery heart rate and a two-minute recovery heart rate. Athletes should be under five minutes.

Average RPMs: about 63–64 should get the numbers under five

One-minute recovery: 25 BPM is good

Two-minute recovery: 50 BPM

Workout 2: 10/20s

10/20s are a nice introduction to interval work. This is actually programmed into the Assaults so all you have to do is push a button. These are done in sets of eight sprints, where each set takes four minutes.

Pace: Use 120% of the average RPMs from the previous two-mile test. This means if an athlete averaged 60 RPMs, he or she would sprint at 72 RPMs.

Rest: Plan on one minute between sets or until the heart rate drops to 60% of the age-adjusted max.

Sets: two or three

Total time: about 15 minutes

Workout 3: Time Trials

Similar to the two-mile MAS test, we'll get times for three miles, five miles, seven miles and, if you have some masochist in you, 10 miles. Pick a distance, have your athlete ride it, then record it.

Pace: Try to hold a pace five seconds over the athlete's mile time from the two-mile MAS test.

Workout 4: 20/10, 10/20

This is the beginning of Tabatas. The Tabata protocol calls for 20 seconds all-out, followed by 10 seconds of rest, where the athlete will barely move the pedals. We do one set of 8 x 20/10 (four minutes) and then follow with a 8 x 10/20 set (four minutes).

Rest: Use one minute between sets or until the heart rate drops to 60% of the age-adjusted max.

Total time: about 15 minutes

Pace: 110% of MAS for 20/10, 120% for 10/20

Workout 5: Descending Ladder—
.6 mile, .5 mile, .4 mile, .3 mile, .2 mile, .1 mile

In this ride, have your athlete try to hold 110% of the MAS pace for every interval. In my case, my MAS is 64 RPMs, so I try to ride each interval over 70 RPM.

Rest: Use one minute between sets or until the heart rate drops to 60% of the age-adjusted max.

Total time: about 10–12 minutes

Workout 6: Three Periods
(I love this one for our hockey players.)

20/10 x 8, Rest one minute
30/30 x 4, Rest one minute
10/20 x 8
Total: 14 minutes

Strength and Conditioning Coaching

20/10s are 110% of MAS; 30/30s are also 110%; 10/20s are 120%. This means if the MAS was 60, the speeds would be 66, 66 and 72 RPMs.

Workout 7: Descending Calorie Ladder— 50 calories, 40 calories, 30 calories, 20 calories, 10 calories

Here we'll ride at 110% of MAS for each calorie count. The rest period is one minute between rides, for an approximate total time of 12 minutes.

Workout 8: .4 miles x 5

Have your athletes ride .4 miles in under one minute, then rest one minute or until the heart rate hits 60%.

Total time: eight minutes

Workout 9: 30/30 x 10

Have your athletes ride 30 seconds on, 30 seconds off for 10 reps.

Total time: 10 minutes

Workout 10: 15 seconds on, 15 seconds off

This one is to ride 15 seconds on, 15 seconds off for 10 reps.

Total time: five minutes

Workout 11: 100 Calories for Time

We have the athletes just go for it here. Athletes will break seven minutes.

Workout 12: Modified Death by Bike— This is a modification of a CrossFit bike workout

100 calories for time
Rest two minutes
50 calories for time
Rest two minutes
25 calories for time

14–15 calories per minute is a pretty good pace. My best is slightly under seven minutes for 100, 3:20 for 50 and 1:40 for 25.

This is a tough one.

Want to Stink This Winter? I Have the Answer

Catchy title? This is for all parents who are trying to help their kids get in shape for a winter sport. I spoke with a mom the other day who inspired me to write this. There's a saying I use often in my talks; it's the title of this article.

If you want a child to perform poorly this winter, I have the answer: cross country. I've had countless parents over the years tell me they can't figure out why little Janie or Johnny had such a bad spring season. They worked so hard in the fall, running all those miles.

Let's get some facts straight. First, there are no team sports where you run for miles at a time. Although athletes may cover miles in a game, those miles are done as a series of sprints interspersed with a series of walks or jogs. In the case of a more rare sport like ice hockey, athletes sprint, leave the playing surface and then sit down. But running long distances doesn't prepare us well to run short distances.

There's a concept in sports called "sport-specific training." The idea basically means that from a conditioning perspective, the best way to condition for a sport is to mimic the energy systems of that sport. If the sport is sprint, jog, walk, the training should be some version of sprint, jog, walk.

There's another important but simple concept to grasp here: *Train slow, get slow*.

It's very difficult to make someone run fast and very easy to make someone run slow. If you want to make athletes slow, ask them to run slower, longer. They may get in shape, but it's the wrong shape.

Injuries are another problem with a steady-state sport like cross country. Did you know that something like 60% of the people who take up running get injured? Those are really crappy odds.

Last and certainly not least, who dominates in sports? The fastest athlete! The athlete with the highest vertical!

Yes, conditioning matters, but let's train for the sport. Lift weights, jump, sprint. Gain power. It takes years to gain strength and power. We can get athletes in shape in a matter of weeks. Most kids are playing their sports at least a few times a week in the off-season, so strength and power are much bigger concerns than conditioning.

Don't give the gift of slowness. If your athletes aren't cross country runners, don't run cross country. If you like a nice outdoor run and don't care about speed, be my guest. But if you want your athletes to get faster and get in great sports condition, train them the way the best athletes train. Use a combination of strength training and interval training to prepare properly.

CHAPTER 13
COMPUTERIZING YOUR PROGRAM

Some readers may feel I'm being contradictory by including a section on using the computer to improve program design. Earlier, I advocated spending time coaching and not getting caught up with office work. However, as a strength and conditioning program grows, the computerization of programs become a necessary evil. For this reason, a basic primer on spreadsheets seems appropriate in a book like this.

Using Microsoft Excel or a comparable spreadsheet program to develop training programs will, in fact, allow more time to coach. Athletes who've been tested can be given a prepared spreadsheet containing most of the sets and reps they'll need for an entire workout. This will free you up to do what you do best: coach.

In order to design spreadsheet programs, you need to learn how to enter formulas in cells.

To create a formula, simply take the cell reference (in the case of the following chart, A3 is the athlete's bench 1RM) and multiply it by the percentage of 1RM desired for that set. The spreadsheet will then calculate the weight for the set and automatically adjust the sets if you change the max number.

Bench 1 RM	DB Bench 8 RM	Close Grip Pre 1 RM	Close Grip 8 RM	Incline Pre 1 RM	DB Incline 8 RM	Alt DB Inc 8 RM	DB Press 8 RM
140	45	126	101	105	34	32	27
145	46	131	104	109	35	33	28
150	48	135	108	113	36	34	29
155	50	140	112	116	37	35	30
160	51	144	115	120	38	36	31
165	53	149	119	124	40	37	32
170	54	153	122	128	41	38	33
175	56	158	126	131	42	39	34
180	58	162	130	135	43	41	35
185	59	167	133	139	44	42	36
190	61	171	137	143	46	43	37
195	62	176	140	146	47	44	38
200	64	180	144	150	48	45	39
205	66	185	148	154	49	46	40
210	67	189	151	158	50	47	41
215	69	194	155	161	52	48	42
220	70	198	158	165	53	50	43
225	72	203	162	169	54	51	44
230	74	207	166	173	55	52	45
235	75	212	169	176	56	53	46
240	77	216	173	180	58	54	47
245	78	221	176	184	59	55	48
250	80	225	180	188	60	56	49
255	82	230	184	191	61	57	50
260	83	234	187	195	62	59	51
265	85	239	191	199	64	60	52
270	86	243	194	203	65	61	53
275	88	248	198	206	66	62	54
280	90	252	202	210	67	63	55
285	91	257	205	214	68	64	56
290	93	261	209	218	70	65	57
295	94	266	212	221	71	66	58
300	96	270	216	225	72	68	59
305	98	275	220	229	73	69	59
310	99	279	223	233	74	70	60
315	101						

All formulas in Excel must begin with an equals sign. The formula might tell the spreadsheet that in cell F14, you'd like to use a number that corresponds to 75 percent of the 1RM found in cell E3. The asterisk is the symbol Excel recognizes as a multiplier sign. Don't use an "x."

If you can master this, you can easily develop computerized programs. When using spreadsheets, you'll develop a relationship between exercises to allow the prediction of loads for a large number of exercises by knowing a few maxes.

A Few Tips

You can obtain dumbbell weights for upper-body pressing exercises by using a conversion of 80% from a barbell exercise to a dumbbell exercise.

For example, if an athlete can bench press 300 pounds, he can do five reps at approximately 87.5%. This would work out to 265 pounds for five reps. If you wanted to calculate a dumbbell bench press, you'd take 80 percent of 265 and divide it by two to get the dumbbell weights.

This would be approximately 210 pounds, which would work out to 105-pound dumbbells for five reps for a 300-pound bench presser.

The formula would look like this:

$$=.7 * D3/2$$

You're probably wondering where .7 came from—87.5 times 80% for the dumbbell conversion gives us 70%. D3 is the cell reference for the bench press max. The next chart is provided to show additional relationships between the various lifts.

BENCH	DB BENCH	CLOSE GRIP	CLOSE GRIP	INCLINE	DB INCLINE	ALT DB INCLINE	DB PRESS
1 RM	8 RM	Pre 1 RM	8 RM	Pre 1 RM	8 RM	8 RM	8 RM
140	45	126	101	105	34	32	27
145	46	131	104	109	35	33	28
150	48	135	108	113	36	34	29
155	50	140	112	116	37	35	30
160	51	144	115	120	38	36	31
165	53	149	119	124	40	37	32
170	54	153	122	128	41	38	33
175	56	158	126	131	42	39	34
180	58	162	130	135	43	41	35
185	59	167	133	139	44	42	36
190	61	171	137	143	46	43	37
195	62	176	140	146	47	44	38
200	64	180	144	150	48	45	39
205	66	185	148	154	49	46	40
210	67	189	151	158	50	47	41
215	69	194	155	161	52	48	42
220	70	198	158	165	53	50	43
225	72	203	162	169	54	51	44
230	74	207	166	173	55	52	45
235	75	212	169	176	56	53	46
240	77	216	173	180	58	54	47

CHAPTER 14
DESIGNING PROGRAMS FOR TEAMS OR GROUPS

Until now, we've discussed things in more of an "ideal model" scenario. However, in a team or group setting, ideal is often impossible. Decisions are made based on how many pieces of equipment are available, and what the equipment will be used for on that particular day.

COVID was actually a great reorganizer for us. The necessity of individual stations caused us to improve our workflow. When the COVID restrictions were lifted, we didn't return to our previous setup; we stayed with a pod setup.

For example, if as the coach you decide you'll program bench press on Mondays, your power rack can only be used for bench pressing on Monday. If you also place another exercise in Monday's workout that requires a power rack, you don't have a scientific problem—you have a logistical problem. Athletes would be competing to use the same piece of equipment for two different exercises. The logical answer is to use the power rack for bench pressing and program your other rack exercise on a different day. This affords maximum use of space and equipment.

Think about available equipment and traffic flow versus thinking about ideal workouts. The ideal workout is the one that runs smoothly based on time and equipment.

This process could continue with any start or finish time with groups moving from station to station in an orderly fashion. In this way, all equipment is utilized and athletes don't have to wait for equipment. This is a logistical plan that can work for two-, three- or four-day workout plans.

Strength and conditioning in the private sector, at the high school level and even at the college level is as much about logistics as it is about science. Very often, the program isn't dictated by what you want to do as much as by your available equipment.

In the section on program design, we discussed the merits of four-day or three-day workouts in the off-season. Choosing a three-day program over a four-day program might mean two more teams can participate in an organized strength and conditioning program. The question is always "how many athletes can we process each day based on the available time and equipment?"

We discussed this in chapter 1 when we covered weightroom design. You want to design a factory with a well-functioning assembly line.

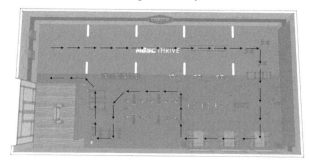

Figure 14.1—Layout and flow— think of your facility as an assembly line.

Coaches must make a decision based not on the ideal workout format, but on which workout format will impact the greatest number of athletes. The "best" workout system doesn't always benefit the largest number of participants.

Even with three-day workouts there can still be logistical issues. Conventionally, three-day workouts would be Monday, Wednesday and Friday and would be total-body workouts. This leaves the weightroom unused on Tuesdays and Thursdays.

For most in-season teams, Thursday isn't a desirable lifting day because many teams compete on Friday. If that's the case, I'd have some off-season teams lift Monday, Tuesday and Thursday. This means that Monday and Tuesday are programmed like a four-day week, while Thursday is a total-body day.

Other teams would be placed on a Tuesday, Thursday and Friday program that would begin on Tuesday with a total-body program, followed by a Day One, Day Two sequence from our four-day programs on the back-to-back Thursday and Friday

165

sequence. In this case, you use all five days of the week and combine programs from the four-day template with total-body days.

This would result in overcrowding only on Tuesdays, but would keep the room in use five days per week. In-season teams would be scheduled early or late, while off-season teams would be scheduled during practice times for the in-season teams.

This type of format allowed us to run an extremely efficient program at Boston University with nearly 20 teams as active participants in the strength and conditioning program on a year-round basis.

Coaching Teams and Individuals

We're strength and conditioning coaches. I don't know if I really like the fancy terms like "performance enhancement specialist" or some of the other names that have been developed to describe our profession. I understand the intent is to give us a more professional appearance.

But the key is *coaching*—I like the term "coach." My father was a coach. Jack Parker, the longtime Boston University hockey coach, is always referred to as "Coach" by all our players. Although I've known him for over 40 years, I've never called him "Jack." In my mind, one of the greatest signs of respect is to be referred to as "Coach."

Learning to Speak "Coach"

It may seem strange, but if you want to be a good strength and conditioning coach, you need to learn to speak "coach." The disconnect between strength and sport coaches is often like a language barrier in a foreign country.

Sport coaches say things like, "We don't want to do football stuff," or "We want a program specific to our sport." Instead of trying to find common ground, strength coaches often battle back at sport coaches by saying things like, "Strong is strong and fast is fast; you coaches just don't get it."

The truth is most coaches don't get it on either side. Sport coaches believe that football players are supposed to be in the weightroom lifting heavy weights. In the non-football coach's mind, other athletes should be running and lifting light weights so they don't get too bulky and lose speed. So, how do we get around all these old-school thoughts?

The simple answer is to learn to speak "coach."

Do you think your soccer coach will respond if you proclaim that when the players get faster, they'll get to more loose pucks or score more touchdowns? Of course not. In soccer, it's winning the 50–50 ball. You need to know the language and culture of every sport you intend to coach.

How about if you tell a soccer coach that hang cleans will increase the players' vertical jump, and they'll be able to dunk? Obviously, a soccer coach could care less, but if I say, "We'll control more headers off corners," those eyes will light up. When I say, "We'll dominate in the box on set pieces," we're now talking the same language. I've said the same thing, but in a different language.

In hockey, coaches say things like, "Who needs upper-body strength?" When I answer, "We do," and then mention that hockey is the fastest game in the world, routinely played at over 20 miles per hour with less padding than football and with the highest speed collisions in sport, they immediately say, "Boy, do we need upper-body strength," and "Mike really understands our game."

If I really want to lay it on thick, I also mention that hockey players are the only players placed inside an immovable ring that creates tremendous collisions with immovable objects (the boards).

I could give example after example of how to speak coach. In women's basketball and soccer, strength training is important because it helps to prevent ACL injuries. Want to get a female coach's attention? Talk ACL prevention. That's the hot button with them.

The truth is, strength training will make her players run faster and jump higher, but the way to sell the strength program in women's basketball and soccer is spelled A–C–L.

When the swimming coach doesn't want the athletes to lift, you simply say, "But Coach, in short-course swimming, at least 33% of the race is start and turn." What makes for good starts and turns? Leg strength and leg power. Suddenly, you know swimming, the coach is your buddy, and the athletes are lifting.

Bottom line is understanding the sport and the athletes you're working with and learning what makes the players and coach tick. Many strength coaches fail not because they don't know their material, but because they don't speak the language of the sport.

Imagine this. You go to France. No one speaks English. Everywhere you go, you speak English and no one responds. Would you be surprised that no one paid attention to you? Would you be frustrated? Learn to speak the sport's language.

If I Was Back in Football Strength and Conditioning

I started thinking specifically about what I'd do if suddenly I found myself back in the American football world.

Here are four things I'd focus on.

First, I'd meet with the staff.

The best way to succeed as a strength and conditioning coach for any sport is to develop the head coach's trust and second, the assistant coach's trust. In most cases, you probably wouldn't have the job if that wasn't the case, but let's deal with the theoretical idea that the athletic director hired you or that you were a holdover. To develop the head coach's trust, you need face-to-face time and conversations, not arguments or confrontations. You might even need to placate a coach in the initial year as you build your relationship.

Second, in those meetings, my biggest sales pitch would be that we only want to change one thing.

I'd tell the coach I want to switch from double-leg squats to single-leg squats. We'd still bench press, hang clean and deadlift.

To accomplish my goal of switching from double-leg to single-leg squat variations, I'd discuss position specificity and injury prevention. It's usually an offensive or defensive line coach who'll push back the hardest, thinking the guys need to be big and strong, perceiving that not doing double-leg squats means less strength.

I'd really emphasize that this isn't the case and that we'd still be pushing for big hang clean and trap bar deadlift numbers. I'd also emphasize the deadlift over the squat, citing the better, more-specific body position with the hips slightly higher, as well as the grip strength and upper-back benefits of deadlifts over squats.

When trying to get through to line coaches, I often discuss specific football techniques (like how linemen are taught to step) and emphasize the unilateral nature of these skills. No one "fires out" off of two feet anymore.

Strangely, line coaches generally agree during the technical discussion, but still push back against a unilateral approach to lower-body strength.

I would also discuss back injuries, particularly if the team has had athletes with weightroom-related issues. Here's where I love to pull out the quote about the best ability in sport being "availability." NFL teams get this, but high school and college coaches don't seem to.

I would also find every video clip I could of NFL guys doing heavy unilateral stuff. Football coaches love the idea of doing what everyone else is doing. Copying success is a way of life in football.

The third area I'd address would be speed training.

I've outlined my thoughts on this in the speed training section of this book, but the bottom line is that athletes don't sprint enough. I'd also be clear about the distinction between sprinting and running. If you don't time these drills, you can't establish what sprinting represents.

In fact, I'd be timing sprints in-season!

Lastly, I would push things like the "Christian McCaffery trains like a track athlete" narrative even though I might not 100% buy it.

Winning over reluctant coaches is like building a case in court; you need evidence and you need to be persuasive. It's important to talk about what you won't change and make the "squat thing" into an intelligent change that will improve performance and prevent injury.

Coaching John Wooden Style

I've spent quite a bit of time reading about how to get better, both as an athlete and as a coach. I've read books like *Outliers, Talent is Overrated* and *The Talent Code*. All were similar and all emphasized a few key points. The most basic concept was Anders Ericson's concept of deliberate practice. All three authors made reference to Ericson's idea of 10 years or 10,000 hours. All three authors also mentioned passion as the real missing key.

However, *The Talent Code* spent a great deal of time talking about former UCLA basketball coach John Wooden and how he perfected the concept of teaching in practice.

The key to the 10,000 hours lies in the concept of deliberate practice. The feedback we provide is a major key in deliberate practice. Practice isn't just

Strength and Conditioning Coaching

a mindless act of repetition, but rather a constant stream of feedback.

The Talent Code author Daniel Coyle notes that:

"Wooden didn't give speeches. He didn't do chalk talks. He didn't dole out punishment laps or praise. In all, he didn't sound or act like any coach they'd ever encountered."

"There were no lectures, no extended harangues…he rarely spoke longer than 20 seconds."

"Gallimore and Tharp (researchers) recorded and coded 2,326 discrete acts of teaching. Of them, a mere 6.9% were compliments. Only 6.6% were expressions of displeasure. But 75% were pure information: what to do, how to do it, when to intensify an activity. One of Wooden's most frequent forms of teaching was a three-part instruction where he modeled the right way to do something, showed the incorrect way, and then remodeled the right way, a sequence that appeared in Gallimore and Tharp's notes simply as 'Wooden.'"

"Wooden's demonstrations rarely take longer than three seconds, but are of such clarity that they leave an image in memory much like a textbook sketch."

"The coach would spend two hours each morning with his assistants planning that day's practice, then write out a minute-by-minute schedule on three-by-five cards. No detail was too small to be considered. Wooden famously began each year by showing players how to put on their socks, to minimize the chance of blisters."

"His skill resided in the Gatling-gun rattle of targeted information he fired at his players. This, not that. Here, not there His words and gestures served as short, sharp impulses that showed his players the correct way to do something.

He was seeing and fixing errors. He was honing circuits."

"He taught in chunks, using what he called the 'whole part method.' He would teach players an entire move, then break it down to work on its elemental actions.

He formulated laws of learning: explanation, demonstration, imitation, correction, and repetition. Seek the small improvement one day at a time. That's the only way it happens—and when it happens, it lasts. You Haven't Taught Until They Have Learned, *authored by Gallimore and former Wooden player Swen Nater states 'Repetition is the key to Learning.'"*

Coaching Kids

Coaching kids is a balancing act. Kids are kids. They should be having fun training. However, at ages 13–15, they should also be learning there's a serious aspect to training.

If you're having trouble controlling a group, I strongly advocate removing those who are most disruptive, or at least threatening removal. The threat of getting kicked out adds a bit of "what if" to the equation. What if I have to go home and explain that I got kicked out of a training session? What if I have to tell my sport coach or my parents?

This "threat" usually gets the message across. You're the boss, and this is a practice. You really have to learn to be "tight, but loose." You have to establish boundaries.

With kids, it's a constant push–pull. Sometimes you're pushing them forward from an effort standpoint and other times you'll pull them back from silliness. With girls, you can be pushing them to try a heavier load; with boys you might be pulling them back from trying to impress the other boys.

Start with simple organizational stuff. Put the kids in lines—and keep them in lines. Always use lines, no circles. Keep everyone where you can see them. Having kids behind you is an invitation to screw around. Call out those who distract the others.

With kids, we want to be light on science and heavy on structure. You can keep them busy as the loads are light and the work is primary technical. Rest between sets isn't nearly as critical as it is with older, stronger and more experienced athletes. I use their energy as a guideline. If they have time to screw around, we're probably going too slowly.

On the flipside, develop relationships with the problem kids. Winning them over is the goal, not kicking them out. Kicking them out should be the last resort.

Develop relationships with all the kids. Learn all their names and ideally learn about them. Do they have siblings? Do they have two parents in the home? Do they have two moms or two dads (more common than you think these days)? Do their grandparents drop them off? Remember, relationships will end up being the best part of coaching. You can change lives for the better.

I advocate the previously mentioned John Wooden-style of teaching for everything we do. This works particularly well with kids. The simple "do this, not that" approach works wonders.

Show them three times while telling them. Give a good demo, followed by the most common mistake, and finish with the good demo again.

Demos have a much bigger impact than the words. Kids today are powerfully visual. Keep the talk to a minimum and let them learn by doing.

Training kids can be the best experience or the worst. Remind yourself that you're the facilitator, the culture creator. You'll get what you ask for. Ask for more.

Writing Versus Coaching

There are many intelligent people in our profession who can write a good program or give a good presentation. However, there are only a few great coaches. The great coaches produce great results. They produce great technical lifters and great performers on the field or court.

I've often been asked what I think has made me more successful than the average person in our field. I don't think I'm smarter or work harder than many of my peers. My answer to the question is that I can get people to do what I want them to do. I make them understand the importance of being attentive to all the details.

The information that follows is information we give to all of our coaches prior to the start of our sessions. I believe anyone who coaches or personal trains will find it valuable.

Key Points

1) Attention to detail: Okay is not okay. Good enough is not good enough. You should be striving to perfect the techniques and movement patterns of every athlete. If athletes can't perform a movement or exercise, you must consistently work with them until they can. Staff members must be consistent in what they're saying and teaching. Athletes should never get the idea that the staff isn't on the same page. Bring up any gray areas in the next staff meeting so they can be cleared up.

2) Remember the Golden Rule, "Do unto others as you would have them do unto you." This means treat your athletes or clients the way you want to be treated.

3) Get to know your athletes or clients. You must know their injury history, training background and a little bit about them personally. You will be amazed at what some true interpersonal interaction will do.

4) If you're talking about an athlete or fellow staff member, you should be talking to them. This means no gossip, no complaining. You must have the nerve to talk directly to the person you have a problem with.

5) Be verbal. Effective communication skills are key in this business. Your athletes will arrive with a diverse range of backgrounds. Some may have extensive experience in what you'll consider proper technique, while some will have none. Provide a steady stream of verbal reinforcement. Be positive as well as negative.

6) Be hands-on. Don't be afraid to put athletes in the correct position. You won't break them. Manual coaching will more rapidly engrain motor patterns. Often, you must create the motor pattern by putting the athlete in the correct position. Both you and the athletes will get frustrated if you talk and they're unable to learn from your verbal cues. There are various types of learning styles, but the best athletes seem to be visual learners.

7) I love for our coaches to be great technicians because many athletes will be able to duplicate what they see. If you aren't a great technician, your athletes will duplicate your mistakes. Perfect demos make perfect lifters. I can't tell you how many college athletes I see who squat

Strength and Conditioning Coaching

or clean exactly the way their coach does. It's helpful to take a USA Weightlifting course. Even if you never plan on Olympic lifting from the floor, you'll learn a great deal on the technical side.

8) The easiest correction in the weightroom is to use less weight. This applies particularly to the Olympic lifts and to deadlifts. If an athlete goes from being able to perform a lift well to struggling with technique, the problem is almost always too much weight.

9) Be careful with humor. What you say can have a strong effect on your athletes. Never make fun of an athlete. Some insecure athletes won't want to train after they've been teased. Some aggressive athletes may take offense to your sense of humor and this may even lead to altercations. If an athlete becomes verbally defensive as a result of your attempt at humor, it's your fault as much as the athlete's.

10) You're in charge, both in the weightroom and on the field. You must teach all aspects of the program. Don't just tell people what to do—teach them what to do. You weren't brought in to be a bystander. If an athlete is doing something incorrectly and you don't correct it, that's no longer the athlete's fault; it's yours.

11) Report all injuries and complaints. Even if you think something is unimportant, it's not your decision.

12) You'll drastically improve your relationship with both your athletes and your athletic trainer or physical therapist if you take an interest in the health of each athlete. If it's obvious a particular exercise is uncomfortable or painful for any athletes, encourage them to get the proper treatment and find an acceptable alternate exercise.

13) When in doubt, ask. You know what they say about assuming. If you don't know the answer, find it out. Never BS an athlete; they'll see through you like glass.

14) Don't take any abuse or backtalk from an athlete. You don't get paid enough to be verbally abused. Deal with problem athletes calmly and politely, but bring the behavior to the attention of the head coach immediately.

Technique Points

1) Technique always comes first. When in doubt, reduce the weight, move a step back in your progression or select a simpler exercise.

2) If the back is flat, nothing bad can happen. Too much arch can also be a problem! You're in charge; you select weights; you terminate sets when exercises are done poorly. We talked about the Charles Poliquin term he coined called "technical failure." This isn't the point at which another rep can't be done, but rather the point at which another perfect rep can't be done. Always stop at technical failure.

3) Be picky. Require perfect form. An athlete lifting the proper amount of weight should have perfect form.

4) If you are unfamiliar with your athletes, start with a weight they can do easily and with perfect form. It's simple to get people to go up in weight and hard to get them to reduce weight. If you're going to make a mistake, make a conservative one.

5) With your athletes who lack good postural muscles, pay attention to technical development. Watch for failure of the stabilizers. Stabilizers frequently fail before prime movers. Common mistakes you'll see are loss of back position in squatting and the inability to return a cleaned weight to the hang position. For athletes with long levers, single-leg exercises may be better for strength gains than double-leg exercises.

6) There's a thin line between conservative coaching and holding athletes back. Some athletes, mostly male, will dislike being told to terminate a set at technical failure. Engrain this concept early. Hold back in areas like deadlifts and hang cleans that have large potential for negative physical repercussion.

7) Understand the difference between acts of omission versus commission. An act of omission is something you don't do. An act of commission is something you do. In exercises like deadlifts and hang cleans, you don't want to commit errors. There's limited opportunity to correct a back injured by poor technique or poor weight selection.

Coaching Points

These are actual logistical points that will improve your ability to coach on the floor.

1) Always coach from behind an athlete when coaching Olympic lifts. If you're behind the athlete, you can reposition with your hands as needed and not be in danger of getting hit by the bar. I like our coaches to be behind the lifter on the right-hand side and to use their hands to draw the shoulders back, to reinforce lower-back arch or to push an athlete forward to get the shoulders over the bar.

2) Coach deadlifts from the side. This allows you to see the back position, which is the major key in deadlifting.

3) Correct small errors. Be attentive to the details. Watch how an athlete picks up the bar or returns the bar to the blocks or rack. A good set is often spoiled by the athlete losing back position when returning the bar.

4) Constantly reinforce.

5) For explosive exercises, athletes should start and land in the same position. The inability to land in the start position indicates an exercise is too difficult or the athlete lacks eccentric strength, or both.

Administrative Concerns

1) When you're busy, make sure your athletes know who's up next and at what weight. Don't socialize with the athletes and don't let them socialize with each other. If you have a group of three or four, they should all be working as spotters or loaders.

2) Make your athletes put weights away correctly. Staff and interns aren't there to compensate for laziness or lack of attention to detail.

3) Remember, interns are there for an educational experience. They didn't sign on to be janitors or shake-makers. Respect will be earned by nicely asking interns to perform a less-than-desirable task and helping whenever possible. Never think you're too good for any job. The lowest form of leadership is leadership by appointment. Lead by example, not by appointment.

Coaching Another Coach's Athletes

When working in the private sector, one question that seems to come up at the beginning of every summer is how to deal with athletes who train with you at a private facility, but play for a team or school elsewhere. More specifically, how do you deal with an athlete who brings you a program you perceive to be poorly written and says, "I need to do this for school."

The honest answer is that we don't allow athletes to do anything but our programs in our facility. We'll usually begin the process by showing the athlete the similarities of their program and ours, highlighting the exercises contained in both. We'll often say things like, "The big difference between programs is in how it's organized," which may or may not be entirely true. Try not to say anything negative about the outside coach or program. I must admit I sometimes fail at this when I see the programs.

To get around this dilemma, our first question when dealing with another coach's athlete is, "What's your testing?" We always want our athletes to perform well on tests, whether or not we agree with the tests and associated programming. Here, it almost becomes like Combine training. We simultaneously train to get better using our program while training for the specific tests the athlete will encounter at school or with a new team.

The two most common tests we need to train for are a back squat and a power clean from the floor. If an athlete has to perform either or both of these as tests, we train for these "events" at the end of the week. For a power clean test from the floor, we'll add sets of power cleans from the floor to learn technique, while simultaneously working to develop power through our regular program of hang cleans and hang snatches. For back squats, we'll do some supplementary sets of either singles or reps, depending on the tests.

For running, we do the same—we use our running program, but prepare for their tests. We also teach any exercises that are included in their programs even if they're not included in ours.

I believe in our program. And I know that allowing an athlete to deviate from our program in our facility opens the door for all athletes to deviate. This is a slippery slope.

I also realize athletes in college or on junior teams have obligations they must meet.

The key for us is to compromise around testing and not in the training. We must instill confidence in the athletes that our program will properly prepare them to play, while training the athletes to be evaluated by their team or coach.

Bob Alejo, Senior Associate Athletic Director at Cal State Northridge, has a good guideline: When working with someone else's athlete, have the courtesy to call the school, introduce yourself, and ask about the program and testing. This is professionalism. I have to admit to failing to do this over the years and making enemies in the process. Follow Bob's advice and contact the coach. At least you'll have done your part.

On the flipside, don't compromise what you believe in. If an athlete comes to you for an off-season program, do what you feel is best based on your philosophy and your facility. It's a thin line, but a little communication and some mutual respect can help you walk it.

CHAPTER 15
PARTING WORDS: THE MIRROR AND THE WINDOW

The job of a strength and conditioning coach is surprisingly easy. You can copy as much as you want. You have access to the same books and seminars everyone else in the profession has. The bottom line is that some people just care more than other people.

I'm a big believer in the bell curve. Ten percent of the people are beyond help; 10% don't need help. Eighty percent will fall in the middle. The bottom 10% will never read this book. Many in the top 10% have probably already preordered it. It's not because of the writing, but because they realize the price we pay for a book always comes back to us.

If coaching really matters to you, your athletes or clients will be the mirror you use to view yourself. You'll consistently push and teach because you realize *their* success is a direct reflection of *your* ability. In the same light, your athletes and clients are the window through which others view you.

I often ask coaches or trainers to visualize a prospective athlete or client simply watching a workout through a window. No sound, just the visual. Are they impressed? This is the mirror and the window. Coaches, like all people, are always watching and it's a direct reflection of your skills.

I've had the pleasure of coaching some of the worlds' greatest athletes. Inner drive is a common denominator. Great coaches must possess the same inner drive that pushes a great athlete.

RECOMMENDED READING

Kroll, William: *The Development of a Football Strength Complex*
NSCA Journal: Vol. 9, Number 5, 1987

Kroll, William: *Structural and Functional Considerations in Designing the Facility, Part 1*
NSCA Journal: Vol. 13, Number 1, 1991

Kroll, William: *Structural and Functional Considerations in Designing the Facility, Part 2*
NSCA Journal: Vol. 13, Number 3, 1991

McRobert, Stuart: *Brawn*

Verstegen, Mark*: Core Performance*

REFERENCES

Bobbert, M.F.: Drop Jumping as a Training Method for Jumping Ability. *Sports Medicine* 9(1):7-22, 1990, p. 8.

Cleather, D.: *Black Book of Training Secrets*

Cook, G.: 1997. Functional training for the torso. *NSCA Journal* (April): 14-19.

Coyle, D.: *Talent Code*

Epstein, D.: *Range*

Francis, C.: 2000. *Training for speed*. Canberra, Australia: Faccioni Speed and Conditioning Consultant.

Dempster, W.T.: 1955. Space requirements of the seated operator. WADC technical report. Wright-Patterson Air Force Base, OH. pp. 55-159.

Dintersmith, T.: *Most Likely to Succeed*

Graham-Smith, P., Natera, A., Jarvis, A. Load Comparison Ratio in Single and Double Leg Movements

UKSCA's 11th Annual Conference – 31st July–2nd August 2015 - Chesford Grange, Warwickshire

Holler, A.: Record, Rank and Publish, SimpliFaster

Ireland, M. et. al.: 2003. Hip strength in females with and without patello-femoral pain. *JOSPT* (33,11, 671-675).

McGill, S. 2002. *Low back disorders*. Champaign, IL: Human Kinetics.

Richardson, C., Jull, G., Hodges, P., and Hides, J.: 1999. *Therapeutic exercise for spinal segmental stabilization in low back pain*. London: Churchill Livingstone.

Sahrmann, S. *Diagnosis and Treatment of Movement Impairment Syndromes*

Thibaudeau, C.: Theory and Application of Modern Strength and Power Methods [Online] available at www.testosterone.net

Verkhoshansky, N. Depth Jump vs Drop Jump. *CVASPS.com* 2013 web archive

Wilt, F.: Plyometrics – What is it and how it works, *Modern Athlete and Coach,* 1978, n.16, pp. 9-12.

Weiman, K. and Tidow, G.: 1995. Relative activity of hip and knee extensors in sprinting- implications for training. *New Studies in Athletics* (10,1, 29-49).

INDEX

A

abdominal muscles and stability of the lumbar spine 45
acceleration vs max velocity, team sports considerations 140
activation drills as part of a warm-up 43
adjustable benches, value of 22
aerobic demand on sports 151
agility, improvement and training of 144–145
Alejo, Bob, coaching athletes 172
Anderson, Gunnar, back pain and surgeries 75
Anderson, Tim, cervical spine drill 49
anti-rotation training, examples of 53
anti-rotators, stability in the core 45
Assault AirBike, Airdyne
  AirBike Elite, thoughts of 157
  program examples of 155
  workout samples of 157
Assise, Rob, power skipping reference 138
autoregulation, based on athlete readiness 114

B

Baker, Dan, MAS training percentages 156
bands, elastic, use of in training 118
bench-block split-squat, description and photo of 88
bench press
  barbell vs dumbbells 110
  keys to bench success 109
  never compromise on technique of 30
  photos of 39
  see also, pressing exercises
Bergeron, Patrice, Boston Bruin, single-leg cleans 67
bilateral
  exercise and the brain 83
  limb deficit, definition of 83
  vs unilateral training 82
Blatherwick, Jack, University of Minnesota skating coach 60
bodybuilding training, discussion of 120
bodyweight exercises, oversimplification of 31
Bondarchuck, Anatoli, unilateral training for athletes 84
Borzov, Valery, plyometic drills discussion 147
Bosch, Frans
  Bosch Iso's 97
  hamstrings and sprinting 97
  unilateral training for athletes 84
Bosco, Carmelo, drop jumps discussion 147
Boston Bruins, strength and conditioning, coaching for 18
box squat
  history of, dislike of 75
  press-out style, example of 30
bracing, hollowing, drawing in, terminology of 46
breathing
  core training and 46
  thoracic spine mobility and 49

bridging
  double leg, description and photo of 50
  glute and core activation drill 50
  single leg, description and photo of 50–51
Bryant, Paul "Bear", Bum Phillips quote about 19
bucket analogy, fillers vs dippers 17
Bunker, Steve, MBSC Middleton coach 136
Burgener, Mike, program design of 33
Burgess, Frank Gellet, quote from 67

C

Carpenter, Alex. chin-ups with weight 106
Carvajal, Jorge. sprint quote 140
ceiling height, need for 24
cervical spine range of motion, drill for 49
chain-loaded leg squat, description and photos of 85
chains, use of in training 118
change of direction, key component of conditioning 154
chin-up, photos of 41
chop and lift patterns
  descriptions and photos of 53
  dynamic, description and photos of 56
  transverse chop, description and photo of 56
  see also, half-kneeling and in-line
Ciroslan, Dragomir, US weightlifting coach 95
Clark, Ken, max velocity work 141
clean blocks, value for hang cleans 22
cleans, see hang cleans
Cleather, Dan
  author, The Little Black Book of Training Wisdom 113
coaching
  athletes of other coaches 171
  compromising on technique 30
  finishing prep work early 30
  good programs vs bad programs 29
  key points of 169
  logistics of 171
  sport coaches vs s&c coaches 166
  when coaching alone 29
Cockrell, Lee, quote from
  author, Creating Magic 69, 82
compensation patterns, affect on core training 43
computerization of programs 161
conditioning
  Assault AirBike, Airdyne, program examples 155
  change of direction training 154
  evaluation of 150
  heart rate monitor, use of 153
  overview of changes in coaching of 149
  sport specificity 150
  sport-specific testing of 152

Strength and Conditioning Coaching

Cook, Gray
  bridging drill 51
  chop and lift patterns 53, 56
  joint-by-joint approach 48
  motor control concept 48
  program design, guidance of 29
  reactive neuromuscular training concept (RNT) 81
  strength to dysfunction reference 30, 73
Cook, Jill
  avoiding patella-femoral pain from jumping 147
  physical therapist, knee pain expert 77
  podcast interview reference 148
Copenhagen planks, description and photos of 57
core training
  brace, hollow, draw in 46
  breathing and 46
  overview of 38, 43
  quadruped draw-in 46
Cosgrove, Alwyn
  training business article, reference to 18
  undulating periodization 114
Coyle, Daniel, John Wooden insights 168
cross-body reach, reinforcing stability 92
cross country, detriments of 159
CrossFit, training system discussion 119
Cross, Matt
  determining loads for sled sprints 65
  sled training discussion 142

D

deadlift
  kettlebell variation, description and photos of 79
  one-dumbbell, single-leg, straight-leg deadlift 102
  reaching single-leg straight-leg, value of 102
  single-leg straight-leg description and photo of 98
  single-leg straight-leg, value of 101
  single-leg, two-arm, straight-leg deadlift 103
  straight-leg or Romanian, difficulties with 101
  trap bar, description and photo of 70, 79
  vs squat 69
depth jumps, discussion of 147
DeRosa, Carl, functional anatomy, understanding of 45
designing and equipping a facility
  adjustable benches 22
  blocks for hang cleans 22
  ceiling height needs 24
  concrete or block walls, need of 25
  dumbbell incremental needs 25
  equipment list, planning of 23
  equipment usage and traffic flow 21
  facility layout for teams or groups 165
  half-racks with connectors, need for 22
  inlaid platforms 23
  lighter Olympic bars, need of 26
  lighting needs 25
  mirror height off the floor 25
  Olympic bars, space needed for 25

designing and equipping a facility *continued*
  planning the weights section 22
  space needed per person 24
  sprint space 21
  turf space needs 21
  weight plate needs 25–26
designing a program, *see program design*
Dietz, Cal, TriPhasic training concept 37
double-leg training vs single-leg training
  muscular differences between 82
Doyle, Chris, programming reference 114
Drake, Daz, single-leg squat standards 84
dumbbell row
  description and photos of 106
  photos of 40
  variations of 107
dumbbells, incremental needs 25

E

eccentric training
  vs concentric training 37
  vs tempo 37
ectomorphic athletes, programming for 37
Eichel, Jack, fly-in times 140
Epstein, David
  author of Range 47
  undiscovered connections concept 84
equipment list, sample 23
Ericson, Anders, deliberate practice, concept of 167
Essential Eight, The
  8 drills everyone should do 48
exercise selection
  concepts of 33
  machines, choices and limitations of 36
explosive exercises
  hang clean alternatives 64
  hang cleans 60
  jump squat 66
  number of repetitions of 36
  Olympic lifts 60
  order of in programming 36
  snatch, variations of 66
  trap bar jump 65
explosive training, overview of 59

F

facility layout for teams or groups 165
Falsone, Sue
  diaphragm and 47
  t-spine mobility 48
Ferrugia, Jason
  programming for "hardgainers" 37
  training business article, reference to 18
first step vs first push 146
Fleming, Wil,
  author *Velocity-Based Training for Weightlifting* 68

180

Index

floor slides
    activation drill 52
    photo of 52, 74
fly-ins
    affect on times 139
    flying 10s, use and examples of 99
    progressions of 138
football, strength and conditioning of 167
foot speed, fast feet vs agility in relation to speed 145
Foran, Bill, football, energy demands of 153
Francis, Charlie
    oxygen uptake vs sprint performance 152
    reverse leg press 98, 143
    sprint training 151
    Training System book reference 13
Freidman, Craig, slide board lunge pattern 90
Frenn, George, box squat quote 75
front-loaded vertical tibia split-squat
    description and photos of 88
front squat, hands-free, photo of 64

G

Gabbett, Tim, research on sprint distance 97
Gambetta, Vern
    Building the Complete Athlete course 67
    responsibility for injuries in program design 35
Garhammer, John, linear periodization reference 115
Gladwell, Malcolm, *Outliers* book reference 18
glute activation, inability as related to injuries 43
gluteal amnesia, injury syndromes of 43
glute-ham raise, description and use of 97
goblet squats
    coaching tips 78
    to a low box 78
    vs split squats 30
Gray, Gary
    knee pain approach 81
    patella tracking, bones vs nerves 82
Griffith, Vernon, quote from 69

H

half-kneeling chops and lifts
    descriptions and photos of 53–55
half-racks with connectors, key to facility design 22
hamstrings, as stabilizers and hip extensors 96
hamstring injuries
    as related to poor glute function 96
    strains, as related to poor glute max activation 43
hang cleans
    alternatives to 64
    as a power development exercise 60
    photos of 39, 62
    teaching checklist 63
    value of clean blocks 22
    vs cleans from the floor 60
hang clean to bodyweight relationship, table of 63
hang snatch to bodyweight relationship, table of 63

Hartmann, Anna, neck range of motion cue 49
Hartmann, Bill, periodization, explanation of 113
Hatfield, Fred
    author, *Science of Powerlifting* 68
    pressing suggestions 110
    program design of 33
    Russian peaking cycle 130
heart rate monitor, value of for conditioning 153
heel lift, single-leg squat and 92
Helms, Eric, autoregulation explanation 114
Hepburn, Doug, pressing recommendations 110
high-intensity programming
    training system discussion 119
high intensity training (HIT), discussion of 120
hip-dominant exercises
    concept of 39
    explanation and examples of 94
hip extension
    straight or bent leg exercises 99
    target of, differences in 100
hip mobility vs lumbar stability 45
hip pain
    hamstrings and 44
    related to gluteal activation 43
hip stabilization, using cross-body reaching 92
hip thrust
    bilateral vs unilateral 39
    shoulders on bench hip lift variation 98
Hodges, Paul
    spine stabilization strategies 46
    Therapeutic Exercises for Spinal Segmental Stabilization 46
Holler, Tony
    flying 10s, times for 138
    max velocity vs acceleration 140
    quote from 16
    Record, Rank and Publish article 135–136
    research on training volume 97
    sprint training, progressive variation, rules for 137
    timing and recording weekly 99
hops, discussion and photo of 147
horizontal pressing 40
    bench press discussion 108
horizontal pulling 40
    dumbbell row 106
    force transmission in rows 106
horizontal vs vertical pressing and pulling 41
Hruska, Ron, Postural Restoration Institute creator 45

I

injuries
    does it hurt? 137
    pain vs discomfort 137
injury reduction
    program design, minimize risk 34
    vs prevention 16, 35
in-line pitcher's chop
    description and photos of 55

Strength and Conditioning Coaching

in-season training 129–132
internship, what to look for during 19
interval training, knee pain during 154
interviews, what to look for during 20
Ireland, Mary Lloyd, et al, knee pain research 81
isometric holds, discussion of 37

J

Jackson, Phil, coaching success of 19
Janda, Vladimir
    diagonal patterns reference 54
    hamstrings, synergistically dominant 96
    posterior-chain description 95
John, Dan
    foreword 11
    quote from 19
Jones, Arthur, Nautilus, founder of 120
Jones, Rusty
    Indianapolis Colts sports performance coach 18
    Super Bowl, team of 19
Josse, Cam
    referral to JB Morin, trap bar jumps 65
    sled training discussion 142
    sled training for speed, quote 143
Jovanovic, Mladen, author, *Strength Training Manual* 71
Jull, Gwendolen, author
    Therapeutic Exercises for Spinal Segmental Stabilization 46
jump squat, description and photo of 66

K

Kazmarski, Brad, bottom-up position 86
Kenn, Joe, explosive exercises, order of in programming 36
kettlebell cleans or snatches, alternatives to hang cleans 64
kettlebell deadlift, description and photos of 79
kids, training of 117, 168
    initial training of 31
King, Ian
    tempo in training 37
    time under tension 38
knee-dominant exercises, concept of 39
knee pain
    as related to hip weakness 81
    related to poor gluteal activation 43
    squatting and 77
Knott, Dorothy
    proprioceptive neuromuscular facilitation 54
Komi, Pavo, drop jump discussion 147
Kroll, Bill
    bilateral deficit research by 83
    NSCA Journal facility design articles 24
Kuester, John, Boston University basketball coach 18

L

ladder drills, discussion of 146
landmine press, photos of 40
leg curl
    variations of 103–104

leg lowers, mobility, core and activation drill 51–52
Leistner, Ken
    abbreviated workouts of 109
    high intensity training (HIT) 120
    program design of 33
    The Steel Tip, program design of 29
lifting gloves, use of 26
lighting, need for quality 25
loaded power exercises, discussion of 38
Logan, Denis, quotes of 41, 59, 62, 133
low-back pain
    from excessive lumbar compensation 43
    relationship with shoulder mobility 74
lower-body training, bilateral vs unilateral squats 73
lumbar stability, vs hip mobility 45
lunges
    inner thigh soreness 76
    slideboard lunge, description and photo of 89
    variations of 93

M

Mann, Bryan, sprint speed formula 136
Marcello, Brandon, overtraining vs under-recovered 61
Martinez, Tom, quote from 19
maximum aerobic speed (MAS), speed testing 156
maximum oxygen consumption (max VO_2)
    measuring aerobic capacity 150
McGill, Stuart
    core and abdominal muscles analogy 44
    drawing in or hollowing 46
    functional anatomy, understanding of 45
    gluteal amnesia 43
    program design, guidance of 29
    spine stabilization strategies 46
    split-squat controversy 86, 87
McMillan, Stu
    speed development, appreciation reference 133
McRobert, Stuart
    abbreviated workouts of 109
    HARDgainer publisher 115
    high intensity training (HIT) 120
    microplates, working with 115
    overtraining thoughts 110
    programming for "hardgainers" 37
micro plates, benefits of 115
Miller, Al, Super Bowl, team of 19
mini band walks, activation drill 52
minimum effective dose, striving for 16
mirror height off the floor 25
mithridatism, definition of in terms of timed sprints 99
mobility drills, 8 essentials of activation 48
Morin, JB
    research on sprinting and hamstring strains 97
    sled training discussion 142
    sprinting for injury prevention 99
    trap bar jumps vs sled sprinting 65

Index

Morris, Buddy, training on Mondays, quote from 123
multi-joint exercises, order of in programming 36
Murphy, Tim, Harvard football coach 18
Murray, Bob, hockey agent 18
muscle fiber discussion 152
Myers, Thomas
    adductor magnus, fourth hamstring concept 76
    author, *Anatomy Trains* 54

N

Natera, Alex
    single-leg strength research 84
    split-stance exercises 86
neck mobility, cervical spine range of motion 49
neck rotation drill, photos of 49
Neeld, Kevin, torso "bowl" analogy 50
neuromuscular system, re-education of 48
Nordics
    isos, negatives of, photo of 97
    rebranded exercises 39

O

Oliver, Jeff, strength & conditioning coach, Holy Cross 67
Olson, Jeff, author, *Slight Edge* 129
Olympic bars
    lighter bars, need for 26, 31
    space needed for 25
Olympic lifting
    high reps in 60
    order of in programs 36
    order of teaching 62
    overview of 59
    single-leg, description of 67
    supervision of 60
overhead pressing, standards for 71

P

Pandolfo, Jay, Boston University head coach 85
Parker, Jack, coach at Boston University 60, 166
Parker, Johnny, Super Bowl, team of 19
patella tracking, is this possible? 82
pelvic stabilizers, illustration of 82
Pendlay, Glenn
    Pendlay position one description 64
    starting from position one 62
performance, improvement of, program design for 35
Perform Better
    balance beams 54
    early clinics, speaker for 18
    half-racks from 23
    Safety Toner Loops 52
    Sandbag Roll 98
    Summit reference, Dan John's foreword 11
periodization
    concepts of 113
    undulating model (Poliquin) 117

Pfaff, Dan
    quote from 67, 134
    sprinting, ground vs bike sprints 138
    story of coaching in high school athletics 149
Phillips, Bum, quote about "Bear" Bryant 19
physiological testing, vs performance variables 150
Pilates Reformer, used to strengthen the glute medius 57
pistol squat, vs single-leg squat 91
Pitino, Rick, Boston University basketball coach 18
platforms, inlaid, value of 23
plyometrics, discussion and phases of 146
Poirier, Chris
    acknowledgements, supporter of 9
    Perform Better clinic, speaker for 18
Poliquin, Charles
    alternating volume and intensity 114
    periodization article 114
    technical failure 30, 119
    tempo in training 37
    time under tension 38
    undulating periodization model 117
    varying an exercises without changing 105
Porterfield, James, functional anatomy, understanding of 45
post-activation potentiation *(PAP)*, description of 61
Postural Restoration Institute *(PRI)*
    appreciation for 45
    breathing and stabilization 46
    bridging cues 50
PowerBlock and SportBlock, useful in home gym setups 26
Powers, Christopher, single-leg stability research 81
power skipping, use of in speed development 138
pressing exercises, bench press discussion 108
press-out squat, photo of 76
program design
    as athletes age 34
    concepts of 33
    ectomorphic athletes, volume for 37
    essential components of 38
    horizontal vs vertical pressing and pulling 41
    isometric and eccentric training, discussion of 37
    minimize injury risk 34
    non-contact injuries and 44
    objectives of 34
    optimal rep counts 36
    overview of 29
    teams or group programs 165
    tempo in training 37
    time constraints 37
    time under tension 38
    TriPhasic training, discussion of 37
progressive resistance exercise (PRE)
    simple method of programming for beginners 115
proprioceptive neuromuscular facilitation (PNF)
    description and use of 54
pulls, *see upper-body pulling*

Q

quotes
  Al Vermeil 114
  Buddy Morris 123
  Bum Phillips 19
  Burgess, Frank Gellet 67
  Cam Josse 143
  Charlie Munger 17
  Daniel Coyle 168
  Dan Pfaff 67, 134
  Denis Logan 41, 59, 133
  Eric Helms 114
  George Frenn 75
  Gray Cook 30
  Gunnar Anderson 75
  Harrington Emerson 117
  Henry Ford 83
  James Taylor 17
  Jorge Carvajal 140
  Lee Cockrell 69
  Louie Simmons 75
  Martin Rooney 15
  Mike Boyle 59
  Schopenhauer, Arthur 80
  Shirley Sahrmann 44, 45, 47, 96
  Simon Sinek 83
  Theodore Roosevelt 19
  Tom Martinez 19
  Tony Holler 16
  Vernon Griffith 69
  Voltaire 15

R

rack system, multi-use, yields of 22
reaching single-leg SLDL
  cross-body reach regression 102
  description and photo of 102
reactive neuromuscular training (RNT)
  example and photo of 81
rear-foot-elevated split-squat
  description and photos of 88
  MBSC use of 86
  photo of 39
recommended reading
  Anatomy Trains, Thomas Meyers 54
  Back Mechanic, Stuart McGill 44
  Black Book of Training Secrets, Christian Thibaudeau 37
  Bridging the Gap from Rehab to Performance, Sue Falsone 48
  Diagnosis and Treatment of Movement Impairment
      Shirley Sahrmann 44
  How to Win Friends and Influence People, Dale Carnegie 20
  James Porterfield and Carl DeRosa on functional anatomy 45
  John Maxwell (any) 20
  Low Back Disorders, Stuart McGill 44
  Outliers, Malcolm Gladwell 18
  Range, David Epstein 47
  Stephen Covey (any)

recommended reading *(continued)*
  Therapeutic Exercise for Spinal Segmental Stabilization in Low Back Pain, Richardson, Hodges and Jull 46
  Training for Speed, Charlie Francis 13
repetitions, counts in programming 36
reverse hypers, issues with 100
Richardson, Carolyn, author
  Therapeutic Exercises for Spinal Segmental Stabilization 46
ring row, modified, upper pull variation 31
Robbins, Paul, measuring conditioning 150
Rollga foam roller, thoracic mobility drill 48
Romanian deadlift, difficulties of 101
Rooney, Martin, quote from 15
Ross, Barry
  author, *Underground Secrets of Faster Running* 69
Russian peaking cycle, modified for in-season 131

S

Safety Toner Loops, use and photo of 52
Sahrmann, Shirley
  glute function and hip pain 43
  injury and synergist weakness 97
  lift pattern reference 54
  primary role of abdominal muscles 45
  quotes from 44, 47, 96
Samozino, Pierre
  determining loads for sled sprints 65
  sled training discussion 142
sandtube, as used with squatting 85
Schaus, Molly, single-leg barbell snatch 67
Schopenhauer, Arthur, quote from 80
Schroeder, Jay, isometric holds, discussion of 37
set and rep schemes, choosing a system of training 113
shoulder mobility, relationship to low-back pain 74
shuttle runs, examples of 154
side plank, Copenhagens as a progression 57
Simmons, Louie
  box squat quote 75
  contributions and discussion of 118
Sinek, Simon, author, *Start with Why* 33, 83
single-joint exercises, need for in programming 36
single-leg exercises
  lunge variations and 93
  single-leg straight-leg deadlift 39, 101
  single-leg, two-arm straight-leg deadlift 103
single-leg squat
  description and photos of 90
  progressions of 94
  step-down, progression of 94
  teaching progression of 92
  vs pistol squat 91
  with cross-body reach, photo of 92
  with heel lift 92
single-leg stability, development of 80
single-leg strength, as a key for injury reduction 82
sled push
  horizontal push, description and photo of 98

Index

sled sprints
  as a power exercise 138
  determining loads for 65
sled training
  detailed discussion of 142
  weighted sled drills for speed 142
  workouts, planning of 144
slide board leg curl, description and photo of 103
slide board lunge, description and photo of 89
snatch, bar and dumbbell, description of 66
soreness, a negative in athletics 97
Spanish squats, description and photos of 78
speed development
  discussion of, comparison to 133
  problems of 135
  speed training mistakes 136
  strength component 136
split-squat
  controversy about 87
  variations of 88
  vs goblet squats 30
split-stance, vs unilateral 86
sprinting
  bike sprints as a substitution when sore 138
  for hamstring injury prevention 99
  max velocity vs acceleration 140
  progressive variations, rules for 137
  space needed for training athletes 21
  speed formula from Bryan Mann 136
  sprinting when sore 138
  timed sprints 99
  timers, sprints with or without one 141
  timing, flying 10s and more 99
  velocity-based training 137
squats
  ability vs inability 31
  ATG, deep squatting 77
  bench-block split-squat 88
  bilateral vs unilateral 73
  chain loaded, description and photos of 85
  elevating the heels 76
  front-loaded vertical tibia split-squat 88
  goblet to a low box 78
  inner thigh soreness 76
  knees over toes 77
  learning progression of 73, 76
  pistol type vs squat to box 85
  posterior pelvis rotation, butt wink 76
  press-out squat, variation of 76
  rear-foot-elevated split-squat, description of 88
  single-leg squat, description and photos of 90
  Spanish squat, description and photos of 78
  split-squats controversy about 87
  split-squats vs goblet squats 30
  split-squat, variations of 88
  vs deadlifts 69
stability-ball leg curl, description and photo of 104
Starr, Bill

program design of 29, 33
  The Strong Shall Survive book reference 13
step-down, single-leg squat, variation of 94
step-ups, description and photo of 93
step-ups, step-downs, single-leg squats
  differences between 93
Stokowski, Joe, speed development discussion 133
Stone, Mike, linear periodization reference 115
straight-leg deadlift, difficulties of 101
straps
  use of, beginners vs advanced athletes 62
strength
  basic standards for 70
  special vs specific strength 143
strength imbalances, contributions to injury 41
strength tests, avoidance of 31
strength training 69
  developing single-leg strength 80
supine progression
  for teaching glute and core coordination 50
suspension rows, horizontal pull choice 40

T

target heart rate, as a physiological measurement 151
technique, importance of 170
tempo in training, discussion of 37
testing
  avoidance of, example of 31
  vertical jumping 61
Theratube, bodyweight squat with, photo of 81
Thibaudeau, Christian, eccentric training, discussion of 37
Thome, Matt
  1 x 20 rep programming (reference to) 136, 28
thoracic spine mobility, development of 48–49
thoraco-lumbar fascia, as the transfer point in exercise 102
time under tension, discussion of 38
training programs
  1 x 20, discussion of 128
  four-day programs, examples of 123
  in-season specifics 129
  three-day programs, examples of 127
  two-day programs, examples of 128
training systems
  autoregulation 114
  bodybuilding method 120
  choosing your system 113
  CrossFit 119
  high intensity training (HIT) 120
  Olympic lifting 120
  periodization, concepts of 113
  progressive resistance exercise (PRE) 115
  set and rep schemes 113
  undulating periodization model 117
  weights, choosing of 116
  Westside Barbell approach 118
transverse chop, description and photo of 56
trap bar deadlift, description and photos of 70, 79
trap bar jump

185

description and photo of 65
determining load for 65
photo of 38
TriPhasic training, discussion of 37
turf space, uses for 21
Tuura, Jake, host of Jill Cook interview 148

U

undulating periodization, Poliquin model 117
unilateral
  vs bilateral training 82
  vs split stance 86
upper-body pulling
  modified ring row 31
  overview of 105
  ratio of pulls to presses 105
  vertical and horizontal pulls 105

V

valgus collapse, hip or knee problem? 82
velocity-based training, issues with 68
Verkhoshansky, Yuri, depth jumps discussion 147
Vermeil, Al
  program design of 29
  quote from 114
Verstegen, Mark
  concept of performance enhancement 69
  diagonal push press reference 43
  isolation for innervation concept 81
  logic train concept 67
  rotary training at Athletes' Performance 54
vertical jump tests, as a monitoring tool 61
vertical pressing, discussion of 40
vertical pulling
  discussion of 41

functional and suspension trainers 111
Voss, Margaret
  proprioceptive neuromuscular facilitation 54
v-stance t-spine drill, description and images of 49

W

walls, concrete or block for med ball work 25
wall slide, description and photo of 74
warm-ups, practical reality in the weightroom 71
weight plates
  1.25 plates, need for 26
  guidance in purchasing 25
  light weight, plastic 31
weightroom rules, need for and list of 26
weights, choosing the best weight 116
Westside Barbell Club
  current, box squat as assistance exercise 75
  original, rocking box squats 75
Weyand, Peter, running speeds and ground forces 142
Wiemann, Klaus, hip extensors article reference 77
Woicek, Mike
  Cowboys and Patriots s&c coach and mentor 18
  program design of 29
  Super Bowl team of 19
Wooden, John
  coaching style of 167
  Daniel Coyle's reflections of 168

Y

Yessis, Michael
  glute-ham raise 97
  program design, 1 x 20 36, 128

ABOUT THE AUTHOR

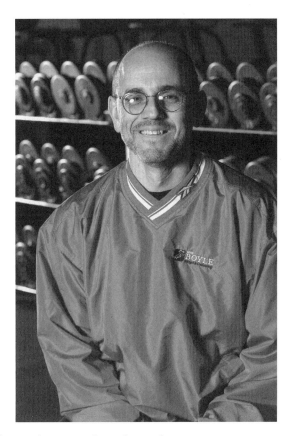

Michael Boyle cofounded Mike Boyle Strength and Conditioning in 1996 as one of the first for-profit strength and conditioning companies in the world. Athletes trained range from junior high school students to all-stars in almost every major professional sport. The business now includes an adult fitness component.

Prior to founding Mike Boyle Strength and Conditioning, Boyle served as the head strength and conditioning coach at Boston University for 15 years. From 1996 to 2012, he continued to serve as an assistant strength and conditioning coach at Boston University, primarily responsible for ice hockey. In addition to his duties at Boston University, from 1991 to 1999, Boyle served as the strength and conditioning coach for the Boston Bruins of the National Hockey League (NHL). In 2012 and 2013, he served as the strength and conditioning consultant to the Boston Red Sox, 2013 World Series champions. He was also the strength and conditioning coach for the 1998 and 2010 U.S. Women's Olympic Ice Hockey teams and served as a consultant in the development of the USA Hockey National Team Development Program now in Plymouth, Michigan.

Boyle has been a featured speaker at numerous strength and conditioning and athletic training clinics around the world and has produced 30 educational products in the area of strength and conditioning.

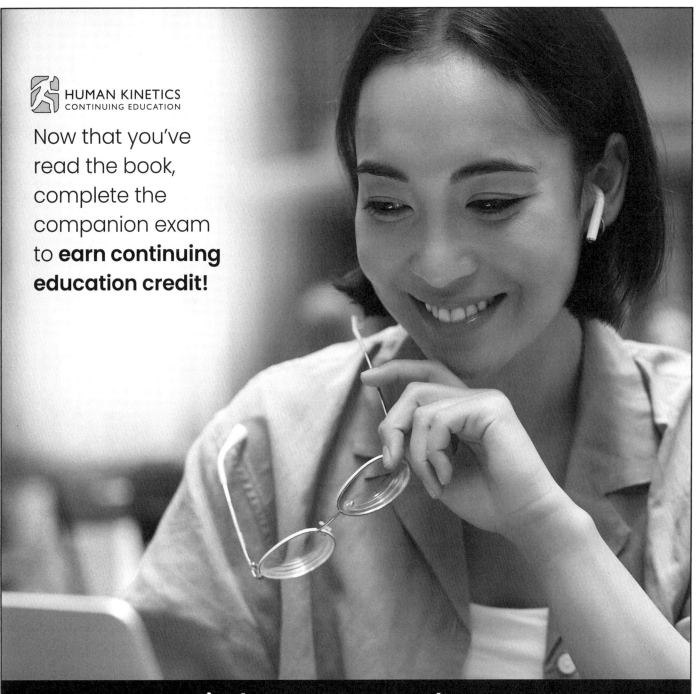